The

ACTION
DIET

35 Practical Weight Loss Tactics as Chronicled by the Fiber Guardian

By Jordan Ring

Publishing services provided by:

Archangel Ink

ISBN: 153079384X
ISBN-13: 978-1530793846

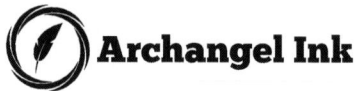

Disclaimer:

The information contained in this guide is for informational purposes only. I'm not a lawyer or an accountant. Any legal, financial, fitness, or weight loss advice that I give is my opinion based on my own experience. You should always seek the advice of a professional before acting on something that I have published or recommended.

Publication of any such Third Party Material is simply a recommendation and an expression of my own opinion of that material. No part of this publication shall be reproduced, transmitted, or sold in whole or in part in any form, without the prior written consent of the author. All trademarks and registered trademarks appearing in this guide are the property of their respective owners.

Users of this guide are advised to do their own due diligence when it comes to making personal decisions and all information, products, services that have been provided should be independently verified by your own qualified professionals. By reading this guide, you agree that myself and my company is not responsible for the success or failure of your personal decisions relating to any information presented in this guide.

Your Free Bonus

Before you begin reading this book, I have a free bonus to offer you. In addition to the information already provided in this book, I have created a printable one-page PDF with ten additional weight loss tactics.

To receive your free printable, sign up for the Fiber Guardian mailing list by visiting:

www.fiberguardian.com/free-bonus

Signing up will connect you with helpful emails about healthy foods, fitness tips, and ways to keep yourself motivated. I also offer even more downloadable content to Fiber Guardian subscribers.

Immediately after signing up you'll be sent an email with access to the bonus!

I am very happy to have you join the family!

Contents

Dedication

I could not have completed this book (or lost the weight in the first place) without the unwavering support of my wife Miranda. She has carried me through the tough times and pushed me forward each and every day. She has made it possible for me to live healthy and enjoy life to the fullest.

Miranda has believed in me since day one. Her support allows me to continue doing what I love, which is being healthy and writing for you!

This book is dedicated to her.

Introduction

Hello, and thanks so much for picking up a copy of *The Action Diet*. I hope you're ready for an adventure of epic proportions!

As human beings we have the capacity for greatness. I believe that by implementing and sustaining small changes, we all have the chance to grasp major success. If we are motivated and informed, absolutely nothing can hold us back.

The purpose of this book is to guide you towards achieving weight loss success, but it will also serve as a means of feeling better, living longer, and improving your overall health. It will provide direction in reaching your ultimate potential through reachable goals and health-promoting strategies (referred to as tactics) to achieve those goals.

The Action Diet catalogs my own adventures on my weight loss journey. I wrote it to share with the world the small changes that were the #1 driving force in my weight loss. I share what worked for me, and hope that these tactics will work for you too.

Did changes happen overnight? No. It took me several months to lose the 50 pounds that I gained while at college, but once I lost the weight, it stayed off. I had my ups and downs, but those ups and downs were gradual and happened over time. I didn't lose 40 pounds, only to rapidly gain 50 pounds back! (Sound familiar?)

I firmly believe that anyone can change their habits and achieve success. Children, adults, teenagers, and even the elderly can benefit from the tactics I will discuss in this book.

This isn't another diet/weight loss book where you do one thing and instantly see results. This isn't another book about a fad diet that will radically change your life in just one day. I'm not going to tell you to jump on a bandwagon and take the rickety ride toward repeat failures. This is a book written by a regular guy who knows that life is a journey, and we need practical steps to make the journey more enjoyable and more fulfilling.

Losing weight is a journey, and it can be an EPIC journey if you're willing to make it such!

The first section of the book will give you an introduction to who the Fiber Guardian is and how he came to be. It will also discuss the first tactic, which is all about focus. I hope you'll be intrigued enough to stick around for the rest of the ride.

Section two covers food-related weight loss tactics, the most important of which is upping your water intake.

Beyond the basic need of water, we all must eat in order to keep on living. Choosing what types of food to put into your body is very important. The choices we make about when to eat or how much to eat directly impact our waistlines and ultimately our lifespan. This section discusses a multitude of tactics that you can use to eat better, such as eating high fiber foods, waiting before filling up your plate again, or trying new foods to keep things interesting.

Along with eating right, exercise is critical to weight loss. Tactics related to getting physical are discussed in the third section of this book. Good news: working out does not have to be boring! There are a plethora of new and exciting workouts to choose from. From yoga to ultimate frisbee to Crossfit, there are a thousand different ways you can get up and moving.

The exercise tactics I list in this book are powerful places to get you started, but if your first picks become boring for you over time, then there are plenty of options listed to replace the activity with another activity. Don't return to doing nothing if that was your pre-warrior modus operandi.

Section four is all about reducing stress and helping your body to calm down. Working out and eating well are so important to weight loss, but stress levels also have a direct impact on your progress. Along with conventional stress reduction techniques, there are surprising tactics that will help you to lower your stress levels.

Section five discusses how to put the tactics into practice in your daily life. I have read whole books and thought "Man! That book was amazing, it has so many good strategies, ideas, and thought-provoking concepts in it!"

But then I ALWAYS wonder, "But what do I do with this information? How will this information impact my life and make me a better person?"

By the end of this last section, you'll be able to put together a solid plan to succeed in your weight loss goals.

If there is one thing you gain from reading this book, please let it be this thought; you CAN reach your goals. There is nothing stopping you, as long as you're willing to put the work in.

Look at Nick Vujicic here on this video (http://bit.ly/1pND1cU). Take a break from reading and watch it now.

As you can see, Nick has no arms and no legs. Yet he is achieving his goals and is happy. There is nothing that can stop you. Nothing.

I have seen countless weight loss programs and dieting regimens fail for people because they quit halfway through or didn't believe in themselves. Believe in yourself, embrace the fact that it takes time to see true change, learn to love yourself for who you are, and start conquering your goals today.

Will you join me on this epic quest for a healthy life and prosperity? Will you slap on some chainmail, raise your sword and shield, and set out on the journey? Will you wage the war against obesity, dehydration, laziness, stress, and hopelessness?

I sure hope you will.

Section 1

THE LEGEND OF THE FIBER GUARDIAN

My name is Jordan and I'm a regular guy. I'm not a gym rat or a die-hard dieter. What I do to stay healthy is not complicated, but it has worked for me. The best part is that it could work for you too.

My life changed when I went for a checkup at the doctor's. I hadn't had a physical exam in quite a while, so I decided it might be a good idea to make sure that I was good to go. Boy, am I glad that I did!

Everything was normal, except for my weight. My doctor spelled it out plainly.

"You are overweight, and you need to start losing weight. However, you're young and should bounce back quickly." She said it matter of factly, with a sweet smile on her face.

She added, "You need to be eating a high fiber diet rich in fruits and vegetables."

My thoughts at the time were, "Okay, duh, I need to eat more fruits and vegetables, everyone knows that! But what is this fiber thing she's talking about?"

I had no idea what she was talking about. I didn't know that dietary fiber was part of the reason I was always told to eat my fruits and veggies!

My logic at the time was as follows:

1. Fruits are okay.

2. Veggies are gross.

3. I will eat neither.

I was pretty clueless! I started researching the high fiber diet. Eventually, I was able to lose all of the weight that I had gained and have been able to keep it off ever since.

It definitely took some time, and it didn't happen overnight. I gained weight over a 4 year span of time, which meant that my body was reluctant to let go of that extra fat. Time was my enemy, but it would also be my friend.

How Exactly Did I Do it?

I went home from the doctor's office that day with a new mindset. I was ready to change. I wouldn't continue on the path that I was on. I would:

- No longer be defeated by my own ignorance and lack of focus.
- Thoroughly research what it meant to be on a high fiber diet and apply what I learned to my daily life.
- Focus on fiber and ensure that I secured my daily amount each and every day.
- Find motivation in the results, which would in turn keep me accountable to continue to attain further progress.

I immediately got my head in the game and researched. I didn't know what I would find, but I also knew that I needed to kick my ignorance to the curb and learn something.

What I found was very surprising. Fiber is found in many healthy foods. It's in fruits and veggies, whole grain pasta, beans, cereal, and even high fiber bars! However, I was eating practically none of these types of foods. My fiber intake was close to zero every day. ZERO! If I had kept this up I would have become prone to diabetes, heart disease, bowel issues, etc.

For pretty much all of my life, I had been fiber deficient! And I soon learned that I was not alone. In fact, just about 95% of Americans do not get enough fiber in their diets every day. This is part of the reason why America is one of the fattest countries in the world, because we are not satiated by the normal American diet. We feel the need to eat more than we should because our bodies are fiber deficient.

I was determined not to be in this 95%. I went to the store and purchased some fruit and wheat pasta, and thus my fiber journey was beginning.

Here is how I started and how you can start too:

1. Go to the store.
2. Find a fruit you like.
3. Find a veggie you like.

4. Buy them.

5. Eat them.

6. Find an exercise that you like.

7. Exercise more often.

Okay, for real. This is way oversimplified, I know. But I had to start with the basics and go from there. I knew that Rome wasn't built in a day and I knew that I would need to be consistent.

I found that it was much easier to start with just a few healthy habits and then add more as I went. I knew that doing so would increase my chance of success in the long run, which is much more important than losing weight right away.

The Path to My Success

It took quite a while for me to come back to a reasonable weight. I had many pitfalls along the way including Netflix binge watching, eating way too much dessert, and an inconsistent exercise routine. I followed no real long term plan, and I know I could have done better.

The great part about being human is that we can read about the mistakes that other people make and learn from them. I tell you these not to ridicule myself, but to laugh at myself. I'm not perfect and I know that I'm a flawed human being. What can I say, it's how God made me!

I will discuss my obstacles much more in depth in the various chapters of the book, but here are some of the more challenging ones that I faced:

1. I focused my college weight-loss efforts entirely on exercise, which is just not enough. Exercise and diet have to work together. You cannot out-work a crappy diet.

2. I continued to drink soda 3 out of 7 days a week. I told myself, "I only drink soda on the weekends! So it's okay!" Well, 3 of 7 days is 42% −− just slightly less than 50%. When I did drink soda, I drank way too much. I wasn't reducing my sugar intake enough (tactic #9).

3. I was battling stress. Deep breathing (tactic #26) and watching my fish (tactic #27) were huge assets in this, but not doing more to combat my stress levels was a huge mistake. This is why I have an

entire section devoted to tactics you can use to reduce your stress levels.

4. I ate way too much, way too often. At first, I would make huge plates of food (honestly sometimes I would just take the entire pot full of linguine) and eat it all. I thought, well, its fiber! It took me a long time to control my portions, and honestly, I still sometimes struggle with this today.

Those were four of my big mistakes. Avoid my mistakes and you'll see success even sooner than I did. Still, I don't promise that you'll see results in any certain time frame. The important thing is to begin making small changes and to incorporate the *Action Diet* into your own daily routine!

Where I Am Now

I'm currently in the best shape of my life, and I'm at my lowest adult weight. I owe it all to small changes and the switch to eating high fiber foods. I enjoy these foods more than I ever enjoyed the junk, because they are part of my lifestyle and more than just a weight loss strategy.

I created the website www.FiberGuardian.com to help people of all ages learn more about the high fiber diet, and to prove that weight loss does not have to be complicated!

I'm the Fiber Guardian indeed. I focused on fiber throughout my weight loss journey, and thus the idea of the Fiber Guardian was born! Mostly because of fiber, but also because I enjoy being goofy and sharing my ideas with the world.

You can succeed If you choose at least five of my tactics and start applying them to your life. The Fiber Guardian recommends it, and do you really want to mess with a superhero!? I sure don't, and I would not suggest that you do. Who knows what other tricks the Fiber Guardian has up his sleeve!

It was an apple that brought the Fiber Guardian to life. A simple apple. *A simple choice to eat something more healthy than a candy bar. This choice led to a hero being born who would make it his mission to help the world make healthier choices. This hero would not only keep himself in the best shape possible, but he would help as many people as possible with weight loss. It would be a difficult task, but it would be one epic journey. Little did he know that to be born meant to be faced with many enemies, the likes of which he could not begin to comprehend...*

Tactic #1: Focus

Let me ask a few questions to get you pumped up:

Are you ready to put the pedal to the metal?

Are you ready for a brand new you?

Are you ready to put feet to your prayers?

Are you ready to conquer your goals?

What is the secret? I will tell you right now: it's FOCUS. Focus is huge for weight loss success because without it you cannot be consistent. Without consistency you're lost.

My Story With Focus

For me, focus was obviously my problem, but I never saw it for what it was. I look back at myself and wonder what the heck I was thinking! The worst time came while I was at college. I was lost in a sea of foods and exercise strategies that simply were not working for me and each year I put on just a little bit more weight.

My mind wanted to multi-task by exercising, eating poorly, and being healthy all at the same time. I gained 50 pounds during my 4 year tenure. I had to do something, and I had to make a change, but I just didn't know how.

And guess what? I struggle with focus to this day! I'm nothing special here, as my ability to focus can be quite suspect at times:

- I can't drive into town and have a real conversation at the same time. I'll just keep driving on the same road and miss any turns that I'm supposed to take. I drive safely, but not necessarily in the right direction!

- My brother used to count after he said "Hey Jordan!" just to see how long I would take to respond to him. The record was 29 seconds...

- Watching a full length movie at home can take quite a bit longer than it should due to distractions.

Needless to say, I struggle with focus, but as you'll learn in this chapter it was the key to my ultimate victory. You cannot succeed without a moderate level of focus. Even a tiny amount of focus will do a lot of good, and will gear you up for long term success.

Increasing focus begins with planning and ends with determination. Deciding that you want to drink a big glass of water in the morning for the next 30 days is a great plan. But it's just that, a plan. You need to focus on following through with that plan to make it actually happen. You need to take action and continue taking action and be determined to achieve victory. The Action Diet is accomplished through persistent action.

For example, during my weight loss journey water was my primary focus. This wasn't easy by any means! I had to be purposeful and intentional about what I was doing. I focused on making sure to increase my consumption by drinking water every morning, as well as constantly filling up my water bottle throughout the day. I had to do this EVERY day. Not just one or two days and then call it good. No change was going to occur in just those few days. I had to focus on the tactic consistently.

Without the focus I gave to this goal I would have been unable to make drinking water a habit. Nobody knows how long it takes to form a habit (some even say it takes longer than the traditional 21-30 days), but truly adopting weight loss tactics into your lifestyle takes a determined desire to focus. As I said before, if you want it bad enough, anyone can find the focus needed to change your life around.

Why Focus Is Difficult

Continuing on the idea of focus, humans were not meant to be able to multitask. Research shows this to be true, yet we always want to be doing multiple things at once.

For example, try playing this multi-task game (http://bit.ly/22LKRlg) and see how you do.

Most people I have seen try this game do quite poorly at first. Over time you can begin to compartmentalize and the focus becomes easier, but not at first.

This is not a true test of one's multitasking ability, but it does show how easy it is for the mind to be pulled in multiple directions all at once, and not give sufficient attention to any one area.

Focusing on more than one weight loss tactic at a time can prove similarly difficult. It's much easier to master one tactic at a time, instead of trying them all at once.

How to Increase Focus

Focus is not an easy thing to improve upon. The following are tips to increase your focus that I have learned through trial and error:

1. Be intentional about learning how to focus better. You have to want to improve your focus and you have to focus on it. This might sound like a catch 22 but in order to change you have to *take action* and decide to make that small change.

2. Learn to take things one day at a time, one tactic at a time. It is much easier to focus on one thing at a time in order to achieve the best results. Just because this is *The Action Diet* it doesn't mean that you have to master all 35 tactics in one day!

3. Be clear about the direction you are heading. If you have a clearly defined goal (#31) it is easier to stay focused and achieve that goal.

4. Ask yourself what it will take for you to stay focused. You know yourself very well (hopefully!). What do you need to do in order to stay focused and achieve your goals? What is standing in your way?

5. Practice mindfulness by cleaning the muck out of your brain. Humans have about 50000-70000 thoughts per day. This is a lot of thinking! Practice putting aside unimportant thoughts, and instead think about what you need to do to be successful.

The Fiber Guardian could feel his mind growing in strength. His level of focus was heightened, and he was beginning to realize his potential. With more tactics soon to be added to his newly expanding arsenal, he begins to see hope on the horizon. He begins to see that he can conquer his foes and arise victorious!

Section 2

WHAT YOU EAT MATTERS

What we put into our body matters a whole lot. There is no way to outwork a really bad diet. You need to put tactic #1 into practice and focus on eating well. It isn't easy to change eating habits (I know!) but you need to realize that losing weight will NOT happen without a shift in thinking and behavior.

For me, I avoided going on a diet like the plague. I never even entertained the thought that in order to be healthier I would have to eat healthier. I just didn't want to even think that I would have to give up the daily donut, sweets, greasy foods, and soda. It wasn't until I wised up and started making changes in this area of my life that I started noticing change. I was losing weight, and it felt great!

Mastering eating habits can be difficult, but focusing on these tactics will bring you one step closer to victory. It may seem like a daunting task, but take it slow and you'll surely come out on top. Someday you may even be so lucky as to wear a cape, have gelled up hair, and really cool green glasses like I do!

Tactic #2: Drink More Water

Don't skip this tactic. It goes hand in hand with each and every one of the other weight loss tactics discussed in this book. The rest of this book is filled with great suggestions, but upping your water consumption is more than a suggestion. It's non-negotiable. If you're not going to do it, don't even bother reading further.

Way too many of us walk around dehydrated.

Water is one of the most important changes you can make to your life; that's why it's tactic #2. After you've sharpened your focus, a good next step is to figure out what your next step is. Finding direction for your goals and figuring out how to accomplish them is no easy task of course, but every goal starts somewhere! Theory and intent is nothing if not followed up with practical action, so choose a direction and **TAKE ACTION**.

I hated drinking water at first. I drank it when I was super thirsty and when I was playing sports, but I never made it a habit throughout the day. A common thought was "Man I feel super tired, I guess I need some caffeine or a candy bar." It never occurred to me that hydration can actually fight fatigue. It should have been obvious, but I wasn't as smart as I thought I was.

My go-to beverage was soda. I loved Mountain Dew, but I would also drink Pepsi, Cherry Coke, root beer, or any other soda you could name. My friends knew of my love for this sugary and delicious nectar of the devil. I would drink anywhere from one can to three cans a day, if the sweetness was particularly calling me.

It's no lie that added sugars are terrible for you. According to the American Heart Association, the maximum amount of added sugars you should have in a day is 38 grams for men and 25 grams for women. I was exceeding this amount every single time I had one 12 oz. can of soda which contains 46 grams of sugar. ONE CAN! I go into this more in tactic #9 (reducing added sugar intake) but on the days I was drinking 3 cans of soda my daily sugar intake was 138 grams from soda alone. YIKES!

I focused my sights on this goal, replacing my soda intake with water. I didn't cut out soda completely, as I still drank it on the weekends, but even just reducing it a little bit would make a huge difference. I later decided to forgo soda intake forever; that decision was not an easy one to make, but it was a necessary one. And it was one I could succeed at because I built up to it slowly and used the tactics to call it quits.

Little did I know that drinking more water would become the Fiber Guardian's anti-kryptonite. (I just referenced Superman there, but the Fiber Guardian is obviously way cooler. Ant-man would give me a run for my money, or maybe even Captain America, but Superman!? Come on man, there are much better superheroes out there.)

Suffice it to say that my superpowers would be nowhere near as powerful as they currently are without staying consistently hydrated. Just like Iron Man is nowhere near as strong without his suit, so the Fiber Guardian is much better off in a state of complete hydration. And so are you.

The Catalyst

Water is the catalyst to reaching your weight loss goals, and skipping this step would be pretty stupid. How's that for clarity? Okay, I will explain it more in depth.

It's actually totally insane how many people forgo drinking water. As I stated earlier in this book, over 75% of Americans go about their daily lives in a chronic state of dehydration! Don't find yourself part of this statistic. Drink more water to start off the day, drink water mid-morning and late-afternoon, and have a big glass with dinner to stay hydrated all day long.

Why do you need to drink more water? What is the reason that this zero calorie drink is so impactful to your health?

Here are some of the most important reasons you need to be drinking more water. This list is not exhaustive by any means, as drinking water has a plethora of different health benefits, but this list will give you a quick idea about just how awesome water is!

- Adding water to your diet is the #1 best way to begin any weight loss journey. If you look at losing weight as a pure math game (which I do not endorse for many reasons), drinking a 0 calorie drink vs. a 200-300 calorie drink 3 times a day can wipe out up to 900 extra calories per day. That's a huge difference, and one that you shouldn't take lightly, as those calories from your drink are most likely all from added sugar.

- Water helps to keep you energized and awake. One of the first signs of dehydration is tiredness and sluggishness, so drinking extra water right away is key to increased productivity. I'm not saying ditch caffeine for water! I think that coffee definitely has health benefits, but there is no true replacement for water.

- Fighting a cold or bad allergies? Water reduces congestion and can help to keep your airways moist and clear. One of the Fiber Guardian's weaknesses is his allergies. If you're one of the lucky ones that don't have allergy symptoms, I can tell you first hand that allergies suck. It's not as bad as being sick, but switching between having to blow your nose constantly and being congested is no fun. Water has been a major help with this for me, and I think it's an underrated way to relieve symptoms of cold and allergies.

- Water is brain fuel. Water can help you to stay focused and keep working on tasks with a clear mind. The brain is made up of about 85% water, so it only makes sense to drink enough water to keep your brain working at peak performance.

- Water helps to maintain normal bowel function. This is especially true when starting a high fiber diet as water can serve to alleviate IBS related symptoms. (IBS symptoms can occur from eating too much fiber too fast, especially if your body is not used to it.)

Take the First Step

Will you join me in adding this tactic to your arsenal of tricks? Drinking water is as easy as going to your sink and getting a glass. Focus (#1) on making drinking more water (#2) a priority.

Use the handy dandy infographic below to find some easy ways to drink more water! It's extremely helpful as a printout for the office or for use on the fridge. Each tip is designed to help you to be able to drink more water throughout the day.

8 TRICKS TO DRINK

MORE

WATER

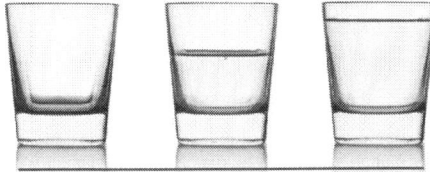

BECAUSE SOME DAYS H2O IS MORE LIKE H2NO

1
Eat a small salty Snack. don't overdue it. but a handful of pretzels will go a long way in making you feel thirsty.

2
Add Lemon or Lime to your water for flavor. As a bonus; lemon & lime aide in digestion.

3
Eat more fruits & vegetables to supplement your water intake.

4
Drink hot tea instead of soda or other sugary beverages.

5
Utilize a Brita Filter, the fresher the water the more likely you are to drink it!

6
Invest in a water bottle you love, and bring it with you wherever you go.

7
Increase your water intake slowly, at your own pace!

8
If you're feeling tired; try a glass of ice water before reaching for your second cup of coffee.

Drinking more water isn't rocket science, but it's something that most people just don't do. I wish I had started drinking water sooner. Learn from my mistakes and take this step right now to make a positive change for your life.

How Much Water Do You Need?

Once you've decided to take the step in drinking more water per day, it's important to figure out how much you need to be drinking!

There are several different ways to determine your daily water consumption. In the end, it's more important to start drinking water than it is to worry about getting EXACTLY the right amount. However, it's good to be aware of the daily requirements to make sure you're indeed getting enough water per day.

1. The most straightforward way to determine your daily water consumption is to follow the recommendation of the Institute of Medicine. If you're an adult male, drink about 13 cups of water per day (3 liters). If you're an adult female, drink 9 cups of water per day, or a little over 2 liters.

2. The second and more complicated approach (but better in my opinion) is to take your total weight and divide it in half to determine how many ounces of water you should get per day. For example, if you weigh 150 pounds you'll need to drink 75 ounces of water per day. This method makes more sense because it factors in your weight. It doesn't make much sense for a 300 pound male to drink the same amount of water as a 100 pound male. When there is more to love there is also more to hydrate!

3. The third and final way to determine how much water you need to be drinking per day is to just drink more water and slowly increase your consumption, until you feel the full benefits of hydration. This is the simplest method and yet it's the most effective and the one that I recommend when starting out. Most of us don't plan on tracking our exact water intake each day and trying to do so can become a cumbersome task. Just drink more water each day, and keep drinking! It takes a lot of water consumption to drink too much, and honestly it's better for our bodies to trend toward too

much than too little! That being said, you obviously don't want to overhydrate, but getting enough water is of vital importance to a healthy and functional body.

Final Thoughts on Drinking Water

Don't think that a little cup of water will turn you into a Fiber Guardian! Hah! You will need to master many other tactics first, young padawan. But if you start with water, you'll be well on your way to finishing strong on this epic weight-loss journey.

Continue drinking water each day and form a good habit. Good habits take a while to stick. It will be tough at first to make sure you're getting enough water every day. Start small and slowly make your way to your daily water intake goals. Remember that everyone has to start somewhere. You can do it.

Focus on water and you won't regret it. It could just be the single most important change you'll ever make in your life. This is a bold claim, but water consumption is everything for weight loss and leading a healthy life. In this chapter I hope that I have stressed its importance enough to convince you of this fact!

Tactic #3: Try New High Fiber Foods

When I was a young child, I hated trying new foods. I would have been content with pizza and fries with a soda to wash it all down for each meal of the day. (Except for breakfast; I loved eating hash browns, bacon, and french toast whenever possible!) I was a pretty pudgy, pizza-nomming kid.

This didn't get any better as I grew into a teenager. I had soda almost every day, and I ate junk food constantly. The options in the high school cafeteria were never very healthy (not that I would have chosen the healthy options), and I ate calzones and chips for most of my meals. My fiber intake was around 0, my sugar intake was off the charts, and I was probably getting very little protein on top of that.

Despite all of this I was never really overweight as a teenager. My height counterbalanced my bad eating habits, and I remained pretty average in size. On top of it all I was fairly active. I played tennis with my dad and my brother, and I was on the tennis team for 3 years as well.

As I told you in the history of the Fiber Guardian, college was the real kicker. Things really went downhill when I stopped growing upwards and started growing sideways. I remained active but continued to make poor diet decisions. The pounds started to creep on.

My unwillingness to try new foods contributed to my poor diet in a significant way, as I didn't buy quality foods to eat when I was hungry. There were healthy options out there that I would eventually love (oatmeal!), but I didn't know it.

Fast forward to today. I will try just about anything! I love trying new foods and increasing the amount of healthy foods that I can have when I'm hungry. Learning to try new high fiber foods was a bold step in the right direction for my weight loss journey.

This initial step might seem inconsequential, but this tactic is truly powerful to get you on the right track to getting more fruits, vegetables, oats, and other high-fiber foods into your diet.

Why Fiber?

At this point you might be wondering **why fiber?** Truthfully, I originally started looking into it because of the direction of my doctor. She said to start eating high fiber foods because I was overweight, and I followed her advice. I narrowed my focus, started eating the right foods, and started heading in the right direction.

Little did I know that a high fiber diet carries with it many health benefits that go above and beyond just losing weight. The decision to focus on these foods happened to be a great one for many reasons! These benefits include but are not limited to the following:

1. Eating high fiber foods helps you to get extra protein (#10), which is great if you're starting a workout routine along with adding fiber to your diet. Protein is needed for the body to recover, especially when lifting weights.

2. Heart disease can be prevented with a high fiber diet. It doesn't mean that if you start eating apples daily the doctor will be kept away indefinitely, but having a healthier diet will most likely mean fewer trips to have your ticker examined.

3. Blood sugar control. Fiber can help to regulate blood sugar by slowing the breakdown of carbohydrates and the absorption of sugar.

4. Increased skin health. Fiber may help to remove toxins from your body that would otherwise be excreted through your skin.

5. Reduction in onset of hemorrhoids due to the fact that fiber moves things along in your system, reducing the need to strain when pooping.

6. Fiber may reduce the risk of some cancers. The research is still out on this one and no decision has been made, but fiber has been shown in some studies to reduce the likelihood of contracting colon cancer.

High Fiber Foods to Try

Listed below are some awesome high-fiber foods and why you should try them. High-fiber foods can be found just about anywhere; that means your daily diet can be fun and exciting! The idea isn't to "learn to like" these foods, the idea is to find foods that keep you coming back for more.

Apples

When starting to look for new foods to try, buy some apples. They are simple and can be eaten on their own or with just about any meal. To the Fiber Guardian, apples are like Captain America's shield, except that they don't block lethal weapons and can be eaten. Apples give you energy to take on the day and defeat Thanos, with or without a team of Avengers at your side.

Apple quick facts/tips:

1. Always keep your apples in the fridge. This will keep them juicy and delicious!

2. Try different kinds of apples. There are a plethora of apple types that all have their own unique taste. My favorites are:

   • Galas

   • Golden Delicious

   • Pink Ladies

   • Honeycrisp

3. Keep an apple on hand at work, in the car, or anywhere that you might need a snack!

4. Pomology is the science of apple growing. Useless fact really, but one you might not have known.

5. The best cooking apple is a Granny Smith apple because of its sweetness. You will find it often in apple pies and other apple desserts.

Almonds

I used to hate nuts. The first time I tried them, I spit them out in the trash, and didn't try them again for years. I think it may have been a walnut, or a pecan, but whatever it was, it turned me off to nuts for a long time.

That was unfortunate, because nuts are one of the healthiest foods you can eat as they are high in fiber and protein, and they contain unsaturated fats which are good for your heart.

Quick facts/tips about almonds. They are:

- High in Omega 3 fatty acids which can help to curb depression and help you to live longer.
- Filled with fiber
- High in protein
- Processed to produce a number of flavors that taste great. Try them all to see what you like (the Fiber Guardian prefers roasted and salted, because he's a superhero and not a squirrel)!

Some nuts to try besides almonds:

- Pistachios
- Walnuts
- Pecans
- Peanuts

All nuts are healthy for you and help to round out your diet. Try to avoid chocolate covered nuts as they are high in sugar. However, if you have to try it with some chocolate first to see if you like them, go ahead! The idea is to get them into your diet. Just be mindful of how much sugar you're eating.

Wheat Pasta

Wheat Pasta is delicious and I honestly like it even better than regular pasta, and it's actually much healthier for you. But should you eat wheat pasta? In truth. 5 out of 5 experts would agree that you should, as wheat pasta is a better option than its counterpart.

You may have read that grains are actually not very healthy, and that they might be slowly killing us. This certainly applies to those with celiac disease, and there is also research that suggests that GMO crops can be dangerous to us when we go on high grain diets. However, on my weight loss journey I had plenty of grains and had no ill effects. I believe that high fiber grain foods were a major part of the reason why I was able to lose the weight and keep it off.

The next time you make a pasta meal, why not try to switch out the normal white variety with wheat and see what you think? I bet you that you like it, and then will rest easy knowing you made a good dietary decision!

Chili

While chili is a meal and not a food in itself, I ate it so much that I think it deserves the right to be featured in this chapter. A chili rich with beans, tomatoes, and spices is a phenomenal way to enjoy food and lose weight at the same time.

You can find my personal recipe here on my site (http://bit.ly/1Scbetg). I've made it countless times and had it for quite a few meals during my journey. Eating chili regularly helped me to get the protein and fiber I needed, and left me feeling full and satisfied every time.

Fiber Bars

Fiber bars are awesome. They are not only high in fiber (duh) but often have plenty of protein and other vitamins and minerals. Here are the two brands that I would recommend. I choose these brands because the bars are low in sugar, high in protein and high in fiber. I like to keep it simple, and these bars taste great as well.

1. Nugo Fiber D'Lish bars – These bars are amazingly delicious and they taste like gold. I've never tasted gold but I don't have to in order to tell you that these bars are amazing. Sidenote – Nugo Fiber found out about my love for these bars and sent me a sample pack to eat and write a review on. You can check out that review on my site by going here: http://bit.ly/1UiDK2e.

2. Kind Bars – These bars are nutty and incredibly good for you. They are high in both protein and fiber.

Ten Other High Fiber Foods

Here is a list of 10 other high fiber foods that I recommend you try. If you find that you don't like some of these foods no problem. Nobody likes everything! Just be willing to try them and you might be surprised.

1. Oatmeal – Easily made and very tasty, oatmeal is an excellent way to start your day.

2. Bananas – Easy to peel and easy to eat, bananas are a great go-to snack.

3. Smoothies with any type of berry – Berry filled smoothies give you plenty of fiber and necessary antioxidants.

4. Oranges – Oranges go with breakfast, lunch, supper, or whenever. You can eat them even if you're so sick you can't get out of bed. Just remember to peel them in your dazed state of mind!

5. Avocados – Add avocados to fish tacos for a cool and refreshing topping while still getting extra fiber.

6. Sweet Potatoes – Perfect for a summertime cookout or a side for your steak. Or if I was being truly honest I would suggest eating them with spaghetti… That is what I did anyways!

7. Raisins – Perfect addition to a bowl of oatmeal.

8. Popcorn – Yes it's indeed healthy for you (in moderation). It is a great snacking food with a good amount of fiber.

9. Broccoli – Your childhood nightmare won't be on anyone's Christmas list any time soon, but broccoli is one of the best foods you can eat.

10. Any type of legume (beans) – Beans are good in chili or as a side.

Trying out new high fiber foods will help you to be able to focus on fiber. Coincidentally, this happens to lead very well into the next chapter, which is all about focusing on fiber! It's almost like I planned that!

The Fiber Guardian can finally feel his belt loosening up! With an improved attention span and a bladder that is constantly full, the Fiber Guardian believes he might be able to finally defeat his arch nemesis; Lackadaisical. He believes that he can finally be free of the clutches of laziness and bad eating habits. This newest power of improved recognition of healthy foods fills him with hope and renewed ambition towards the ultimate prizes: a waistline that would rival the great and mighty Thor and Hulk sized biceps.

Tactic #4: Focus on Fiber

Now that you've been introduced to some delicious high-fiber foods (#3), you're ready to accept the next challenge. Your mission, if you choose to accept it, is to focus on eating a complete serving of fiber every day. This tactic asks you to make high-fiber foods an integral part of your diet.

At its core this tactic is very simple to do. When I started incorporating fiber into my diet, I did it with very little nutritional knowledge (other than knowing that fiber might make me poop better). Luckily for you I make this part of the process a breeze with all of the information on my site, especially my article on 75 high fiber foods. All I did was eat foods that I knew to be high in fiber.

Initially, I didn't worry about how many calories I was eating, or even how much sugar was in the foods. I didn't even factor in fat, sodium, or cholesterol content when making decisions on what I would eat. If it was high in fiber, it was good enough for me. Over time, the weight came off and I learned to love fruits, vegetables, nuts, and grains!

My current repertoire includes:

- Apples. Duh. :)
- Fiber bars for a quick and easy snack.
- Smoothies with bananas and other frozen fruit.
- Brown rice.
- Broccoli.
- Almonds and pistachios.

There is so much information out there about how to eat healthy, and how to lose weight. I know that it can be overwhelming to hear multiple pieces of advice from different reputable sources, and all of them seeming to say different things! I'm not saying that focusing on fiber will be the key to losing weight for everyone, but I do believe it will improve your health and help you on your weight-loss journey.

Focusing on fiber helps you to formulate a better diet, because fibrous foods are typically natural foods like fruits, vegetables, nuts, and seeds. If you focus on fiber, you start to eat better foods as a by-product of your new focus. No wonder I lost weight when I started focusing on fiber!

How Much Fiber Do I Need?

The easy answer is that you need to be getting much more than you already are. It would be a pretty good bet that most of the people reading this book are in the same place I was when I started. I had no idea how much fiber I needed, and didn't even know that I was getting very little fiber in my diet at all!

At first, you need to add fiber slowly into your diet. Too much too soon can be really tough on your digestive system and cause excess gas and bloating. Start slowly, and then increase your intake from there. I recommend taking it week by week and eating just a little bit more fiber every week.

There is no exact science to how fast you should increase your intake as fiber will affect each person differently (and more so if you're currently fiber deficient!). If you want to track your progress exactly here is what I recommend:

1. Week 1: 40% of your daily fiber needs
2. Week 2: 60% of your daily fiber needs
3. Week 3: 80% of your daily fiber needs
4. Week 4: 100% of your daily fiber needs.

Eventually you want to shoot for the following amounts. See the table below to find out exactly where you fall in your dietary fiber requirements:

Age Range (Years)	Daily Fiber Intake (Grams) For Males	Daily Fiber Intake (Grams) For Females
1-3	19	19
4-8	25	25
9-13	31	25
14-18	38	25
18-50	38	25
50 and Older	30	21

The vast majority of the readers will find that they will fall into the range of 14-50 years. This means that if you're a male within this range you need to eventually shoot for 38 grams, and if you're a female you need to shoot for 25 grams.

These daily requirements are based upon a diet consisting of 14 grams per 1000 calories consumed. On average, men need to consume more calories than females, thus the higher daily fiber requirement.

You can eat too much fiber in a single day, but in this case it's better to get too much than too little. Your body will definitely let you know if you go overboard, so try not to overdo it!

Ultimately, your daily fiber requirements should be used as a guideline. The important thing is to start eating more high fiber foods and aiming for your daily goal. I personally never counted my exact per day fiber consumption, and I don't think it's necessary for you to do so either. However, it's important to set concrete goals. Eating an apple a day is excellent, but is only a small part of your daily fiber requirements. Eventually, you'll need to do more.

How the Heck Do I Get Enough Fiber in One Day?

38 grams of fiber in one day might seem like an insurmountable feat, yet it's doable. Even 25 grams for women might seem like a lot, but again, it's indeed possible to meet your daily fiber requirements.

The chart below shows an example of a day that meets an adult's daily fiber requirements. Keep in mind that this is only one way to meet your requirement. I don't suggest following this example to the letter every single day, as it's important to mix things up.

Example Day For Men	The Goal: 38 grams
Cooked Oatmeal	2 Cups = 8 grams
1 Medium Orange	Whole Orange = 3 grams
Turkey Sandwich with Wheat Bread	Whole Sandwich 6 grams
Apple	Whole Apple = 4 grams
Kind Bar	1 Bar= 7 grams
Multi Bean Chili	1/2 cup = 10 grams

Example Day for Women	The Goal: 25 grams
Dates	½ Cup = 5 Grams
Raspberries	½ Cup = 4 Grams
Whole Wheat English Muffin	1 Muffin= 4 Grams
Kind Bar	1 Bar = 7 Grams
Broccoli	1 Cup= 5 Grams

★The amount of fiber per serving for the chili was a guestimate, as it will depend on the ingredients in the chili.

As I said, this is just one example of how to get your recommended daily fiber amount. You will need to get at least some fiber from just about every meal in order to hit your daily requirements.

Start off strong in the morning with a bowl of oatmeal or a high fiber breakfast bar and you'll be well on your way to victory to getting enough fiber to meet your needs. Remember to increase your fiber intake slowly and drink water, and you'll be golden.

Keep Focused

Fiber is healthy for you, the daily requirement is within your reach, and the tools to get there have been given to you. Focus on fiber for long term results and for a well-rounded diet.

I don't even know you, yet I know that you can do it. Why? Because it isn't rocket science. It's simply being willing to try new things.

Keep the focus by giving it your all, and keep pressing on when it gets hard. Things tend to become more difficult right before a change occurs, so keep at it and keep trying your best. If you're able to end the day and you honestly and truly did the best you can, then that is all that you can possibly do.

Tactic #5: Discover Healthy Foods That you Enjoy (and Eat Them!)

Losing weight and becoming a healthier individual is not accomplished by starving yourself. NO! Weight loss is accomplished by finding a diet that works for you that you LIKE (or maybe even LOVE!). Trust me, I learned to love the new foods that I would be eating. I currently think oatmeal is quite possibly the best food ever.

However, I will admit that this is easier said than done. I truly struggled with this at first. The bottom line is that I just didn't like a lot of foods that were good for me. Or, so I thought. I thought of healthy foods as "boring" and avoided them like the plague.

After that fateful day with my doctor, I soon found out how wrong I was! Eating healthy could be fun. Eating healthy could be as exciting as getting a new pair of underwear, or even as inviting as the feeling of a warm towel out of the dryer. Going to the grocery store with a renewed sense of determination and direction felt amazing! I knew that I would be getting certain foods that would be helping me to reach my goals.

I might be kind of a nerd about this, but I found that I loved trying new foods. I had never tried wheat pasta before, nor had I eaten much chili. I didn't regularly eat apples and bananas, although I found that I truly liked them a lot, and I would enjoy eating them on a regular basis.

Keep it simple

It's obviously much easier and faster to go to a fast food joint, order a burger and fries and a shake, than it is to plan a healthy meal and prepare it. But there's a price to pay for fast and easy. Fast food is rough on your wallet, and fast food is terrible for you because of high levels of trans fat and added sugars.

Following the above advice does take more work. I won't lie to you about that. Eating out is easy. But I will also tell you that if you keep it simple, you'll be surprised at how easy it can be to change your diet for the better.

Here are some tips to keep it simple when shopping for new foods.

1. Go in with a plan. Have an idea of what you would like to try out.

2. Buy at least 3 new foods the first time you go shopping. Try getting something new for breakfast, lunch, and dinner. My first time shopping for high fiber foods I decided on wheat pasta, apples, and a wheat bread for sandwiches. Very wheaty, but it was a start!

3. Spend time looking at foods in the produce section. Decide what might interest you, and even look up recipes on Pinterest by typing in _____ recipes in the Pinterest app search bar. You are bound to find plenty of recipes that include the specific produce you're looking at. This is an excellent way to find new and delicious foods that you like.

4. If you like cereal, buy a brand high in fiber and low in sugar.

5. Don't overdo it. Know that it takes time to replace your diet fully. Buy just a few new foods the first time you go.

6. If you don't end up liking the foods you purchased, no problem! You can't know unless you try them at least once.

Other Fun Foods to Try

- Coconuts – Obviously you won't be able to eat a full coconut, but they make a great flavor to add to foods, they taste great, and there are a lot of different ways to eat them.

- Coconuts also have other amazing health benefits including increasing heart health and giving you a quick energy boost. Here are some things you can do with a full coconut: http://bit.ly/25oZ9ut.

- Sapodilla – Also known as Manilkara Zapota, sapodilla is a tropical fruit not yet found in all US markets, but slowly starting to become more common. If you can find one, try it out and see what you think! This fruit is high in fiber at 14 grams per medium size fruit, high in antioxidants, and high in a variety of vitamins.

- Dates – Dates are delicious but high in sugar at 93 grams per cup, so eat them sparingly if you like them.

- Prunes – This food is indeed a good food to try if you're looking for something new. You might like them or you might hate them, but you won't know unless you try. Dried prunes can be found in the fruit and nut section of the grocery store.

- Breadfruit – This fruit's one you might not have heard of, but it can be added to multiple meals. See this article to find out what the heck breadfruit is: http://bit.ly/1RsRKD0.

- Elderberries – Definitely make sure that the elderberries you're eating are ripe, as the raw fruit contains a toxin called cyanide. You can tell when they are ripe when they are deep purple-black in color with a plump appearance. Also be sure to cook them in order to avoid any chance of getting sick!

- Persimmon – Among being high in fiber and high in Vitamin C, Persimmons also have other great health benefits. Make sure these are fully ripe as well before devouring!

- Loganberries

- Guava

- Apricots

Any of these foods will give your diet the extra punch and uniqueness that it desperately needs. Opening up your palate to new tastes and textures is an exhilarating experience, and I hope that you're willing to take the culinary journey.

Enjoy Yourself

The key to adding healthy foods to your diet is to find ones that you actually enjoy. Kale might be one the healthiest foods out there, but I think the texture is kind of nasty. I do not make it part of my regular diet despite the potential benefits of doing so.

Enjoy yourself when you're eating. There are bound to be vegetables that you like that are out there. Squash is delicious. and I never would have found that I like it so much had I not tried it! Some of the healthiest foods out there are ones that you can come to love, especially when eaten in the right conditions.

For example, broccoli and mushrooms taste much better when added to pasta, or cooked as part of a soup or crock pot meal. Some vegetables, like carrots or cucumbers, make great additions to a salad. Try new foods whenever possible, and make sure you're enjoying yourself when you're doing so.

Stay positive and happy as you incorporate new foods into your diet. There is no reason to beat yourself up if you happen to mess up by going back to your comfort foods. Everyone messes up and makes mistakes. There is nothing you cannot overcome. Enjoy yourself, and eat foods that make you happy, just try to make those foods the right ones!

Tactic #6: Make Dinner at Home

Making dinner at home is the way to go. Hands down, without question, without pause or discretion. Eating a home cooked/home prepared meal is the best way to go.

Granted, home cooked meals are not healthy just because they are home cooked. Cooking at home only puts you in the drivers seat. When I was first losing weight, making food at home was a key factor in my success. I ate chili and pasta, added beans and other vegetables as sides to my meals, and slowly began to eat most of my meals at home. I avoided getting fast food nightly, and saved a lot of money as a side benefit!

To be totally honest, I ate so much chili that it was probably coming out of my ears. But it worked for me! As an added bonus, I was able to make enough food for the week, especially when I made my chili. I love eating leftovers, so this was a huge plus for me.

Even if you're not a big fan of eating leftovers, cooking at home can indeed be easy. I'm all about making things easy. First let me sell you on the fact that this tactic is valid, then I will provide you with a few at home meal options to try for yourself.

Why Make Dinner at Home?

Home-cooked dinners offer:
- The potential for conversations with family members which in turn can lead to a happier home life. I believe that families who eat together, stay together. Less tension in the home means less stress and depression in your own life, which is better by far than the alternative!

- Control over the ingredients. Added sugars can be avoided much more easily, and vegetables can be added to just about anything. Even homemade pizzas can include mushrooms, peppers, pineapples, squash, artichokes, or even tuna fish.

- BIG $ savings. The cost for my wife and me to get breakfast usually runs at least 20 bucks when the coffee is added to the bill. This is just for breakfast! If we were to spend that 20 dollars at the store we could buy milk, eggs, oatmeal, english muffins, and coffee and still have a little bit left over. Cooking at home, we could each have breakfast several times. Eating out can be fun, but doing it too often will have a serious effect on your bank statements.

- The ability to save time. This is counterintuitive as many people say they don't have time to cook, but going out to eat can take just as much time when you add in the driving and waiting time. While it feels good to be lazy once in awhile, time is much better saved if you prepare meals ahead of time. Better yet, get yourself a crock pot and slow cook some of your meals. This way, the food can be cooking while you're away at work!

- Trans fats are still prevalent in several fast food chains, along with other restaurants. The best way to avoid trans fat is to see the nutritional value of the items you're adding to your meal.

Home-Cooked Meal Ideas

Some of my favorite recipes are listed below. Try some and see how you like them. Don't be afraid to add your own spices, vegetables, and other ingredients. Experimenting with food can be a lot of fun!

1. Orange Chicken in the Crock Pot
2. Spaghetti With Sausage and Peppers – go for wheat pasta here!
3. Pan-Seared Trout With Italian-Style Salsa
4. Cornmeal Cakes with Smoked Chicken and Coleslaw
5. Shrimp-Pesto Pizza

Any of these meals brings fresh ingredients into your life. Find one you like and try it out. It won't be perfect, but the more you practice cooking the easier it will get!

The Truth about Fast Food

The real truth about fast food is probably one you already know; avoid it on a regular basis. Fast food makes it really easy to overeat and to go over your daily calorie requirements. Many popular fast food restaurants have dishes that are ridiculously high in calories. You can even eat an entire day's worth of calories in just one meal, or just one drink depending on where you go!

For example; if you order a double whopper with cheese, onion rings, and a shake from Burger King you'll have successfully topped 2000 calories with a single meal!

Yikes!

I never would have imagined that you could be getting that amount of calories from a meal, but it's actually possible.

It isn't all about the calories (and I didn't lose weight by focusing on reducing calories) but it's testament to the overall unhealthiness of fast food in general that so many calories can be stuffed into the food.

Additionally, fast food is high in added sugar and sodium, and other ingredients that don't help you to meet your healthy eating goals. Even more importantly, fiber is not the focus of most fast food meals. (Wheat buns at burger king? I didn't think so.)

Making dinner at home allows you to add fruits and vegetables to your meals, and to make foods that do not add unnecessary preservatives and other crap. It may seem daunting to cook, but trust me, over time it gets easier and ultimately it's a lot of fun!

Start by:

1. Researching some meals you might like. Pinterest is an awesome resource for this as it allows you to see the meals first!

2. Going to the grocery store and purchasing new foods.

3. Making a mess in the kitchen and cooking!

4. Inviting a friend over to help, or to enjoy the meal with you! Even better, ask this same person to be your accountability partner (tactic #34).

5. And most importantly: don't give up!

Using his cape as a makeshift apron, the Fiber Guardian looks at his oven with a dual sense of excitement and nervousness. What would he cook tonight? Would it taste any good? Wouldn't it be easier just to go get a Whopper? NO! With a growl he turned on the stovetop and started some water boiling. The succulent taste of homemade chicken, brown rice, and broccoli would soon be on his dinner plate!

Tactic #7: Wait Five Minutes Before Getting Seconds or Dessert

Waiting five minutes to reach for second helpings after finishing your plate gives your mind time to catch up with your body. We were not really designed to scarf down food super quickly. Eating on the go and being rushed can both be reasons why you eat too quickly, but it definitely pays to slow down when you eat. This gives your body time to start breaking down the food and your brain will send the appropriate "STOP EATING" signals to your ravenous appetite!

Waiting five minutes may not seem easy when you feel like eating, but it's really no time at all. It takes five minutes to:

1. Take the dog out for a quick pee.

2. Check your email.

3. Call a friend (but choose the friend wisely!)

4. Take a walk.

How Do I Wait?

Like the other tactics, the hardest part about this is the practical application. Not many would argue that waiting to grab seconds and waiting to eat dessert are bad ideas. But man, the human sweet tooth can be a snarky pain in the rear. It's so hard to fight the urge and to not grab a cookie, hot chocolate, or some other treat to top off a good meal.

It's not easy to say "no" when your trained brain is saying "FEED ME THAT DELICIOUS CHOCOLATEY TREAT RIGHT NOW!" The urge to eat something sweet after a meal is strong and automatic.

I definitely struggle in this area. I love food in general, and not getting a second plate at meal times can be very difficult. There are several tricks that

I use to avoid second helpings, defeat the urge to eat sweets, and to make better choices. It's my pleasure to share them with you here!

Here are some ways to avoid second helpings:

- Train your brain to recognize that the second plate of food is not needed. You already have enough! Do this by really focusing on how much you just ate, and thinking that if you really are hungry, the food will still be there in 5 minutes.

- Savor each bite you take. If the food is really that good, take your time to eat it and to enjoy it! If it wasn't the most amazing meal you've ever had, seconds are not worth it!

- Practice mindfulness. Doing a quick yoga stance or stretching will help you to realize how the food is already affecting your body.

- Only make enough food for one meal. This can be difficult as making just enough is hard. Often, making less than you think you need is the ticket.

- Juvenile in practice, but undeniably effective, try sitting for five minutes after you finish your first plate. Once the timer goes off, make yourself a second plate and eat to your heart's content. After five minutes you'll quickly realize that you're not hungry enough to even bother getting more. The more this works for you, the more you'll start to see just how slow the mind is to catch up to the body's needs!

This will be a difficult weight-loss tactic for many people, but it's indeed possible to limit the craving for dessert. Here are some ways to accomplish this goal!

- Out of sight out of mind (and more importantly out of easy access!). The best way to avoid eating sweets after a meal is to keep unhealthy foods off the shelf. If it isn't there you'll have to go out of your way to meet the craving. You could even freeze your candy bar in a block of ice, similar to how some people freeze credit cards to avoid impulse buys.

- Have a piece of gum right after dinner. This will get something into your mouth right away and will take away the craving for something more.

- If no gum is available, brushing your teeth is a great alternative option. You will be much less likely to eat a brownie if you just brushed your teeth!

- If you absolutely *have* to have a dessert, walk to get it. Walk to the grocery store to pick up a candy bar or walk to the ice cream stand. Walking is a great habit, and the benefits are worth it, even if you're getting a dessert.

- Eat something healthy in disguise. This means eating chocolate covered almonds, peanut butter and celery, or anything that includes a fruit or vegetable. A fruit cup satisfies the sweet tooth, and is really good for you too!

- If all else fails, eat a snack size candy bar. If you keep small amounts around and opt not to purchase an entire bag, eating one or two tiny candy bars can be a good way to not overindulge, but still kick the cravings to the curb. Utilize this method as a last resort option only, because for a lot of us the sugar craving beast that lives inside might just break free in all its glory...

Five minutes can make all the difference. More often than not, waiting five minutes will allow your mind to catch up with your body's needs and you'll start training your mind in a positive way. You'll eventually have fewer cravings and won't feel a strong desire to eat something sweet after every meal.

This is a tactic that has worked for me in the past, but admittedly it's a difficult one to be consistent with. I believe in this tactic, even if it seems like madness to fight the craving for sweets. Try it, stick with it, and keep on fighting. Perseverance is the key to winning the war. Never stop fighting and trying new ways to succeed. Eventually you'll find the methods that work for you, and you'll start to see major results!

Tactic #8: Include Something Healthy in Every Meal (No Matter What)

Picture This for Just a Second

You have just arrived at the family picnic on a warm and sunny day in July. Mom, Dad, and Cousin Pat greet you with a warm hug and smiling faces. The kids are playing badminton and the adults are lounging in the pool. Uncle Bob has the burgers and hotdogs on the barbecue and is flashing the crowd a big toothy grin as if he is the one and only person in the world that can grill a burger.

Since you're on a weight loss program, you're already getting nervous that you'll blow it. Is this the day everything goes downhill?

Walking next to the table full of brownies and cookies of all sizes and shapes doesn't help your resolve, and you're already beginning to tell yourself that it's fine to take a loss today. Your brain is rationalizing its desire for the sugar-filled treats and is already scheming against you.

You feel your resolve slipping even more when MeMa tells you to try her chocolate pie after the meal!

There will be times that getting a healthy meal isn't possible or even desired. Eating healthy ALL of the time is difficult, ESPECIALLY when transforming a bad diet. Sometimes you just want to eat a cheesy, meaty slice of pizza (or a whole pie if we are being honest with ourselves here) or a succulent cheeseburger. I'm right there with you. Some foods are so unbelievably tempting that I find myself giving in.

There are several ways that the family barbeque can go down:

1. You give in to all of your desires, eating three burgers, two servings of potato salad, and most of a bag of Lays chips. Unbelievably you "saved some room" for a hearty slice of Grandma's chocolate pie. You go home feeling pretty sick, and pretty guilty.

2. You muster up an inhuman, steely determination that allows you to resist all of the unhealthy food within your grasp and under your nose. You snack on the nuts that you brought along, and help yourself to a big portion of broccoli salad and a fruit cup. You go home feeling good physically, but sad that you missed out on all of the delicious food. You're also upset at the frown that Grandma gave you when you said that you had to pass on her chocolate pie. Poor MeMa...

3. You decide to indulge a little and have a cheeseburger. You choose to eat just one cheeseburger with a small portion of potato salad, and a big portion of broccoli salad and an apple. For dessert you stick to just one small piece of chocolate pie and let Grandma know that it was amazing.

Option 1 is a complete indulgence, and can set you back for several days, or even stop your effort if you let yourself feel like a failure. It's the easiest path to take, but you'll regret your actions afterward.

Option 2 is a possibility that will hardly ever come to pass. It's a choice that not many people are able to make. It takes a lot of practice and a hardened commitment that takes time to reach, which anyone new to a healthy diet hasn't built up yet. It's very difficult to resist foods that you've grown up eating and enjoying.

Option 3 is a mix of good and bad, yet is the best option in my opinion. It's a blend of eating healthy and indulging to be happy. It allows you to bond with family members and join in the festivities, but it keeps you from going overboard and feeling terrible the following day.

The great news is that Option 3 is accomplished simply by making sure you're getting something healthy in your meal. This means to add a healthy food or healthy side to every single meal—no exceptions.

In the barbeque example, the healthy choice was adding the broccoli salad as a side along with the apple. Nowadays there is usually a healthy option somewhere in the midst of other choices, and it's usually pretty easy to find.

Remember, the key to this tactic is to just incorporate these foods within the meal. You do not have to have just an apple and some nuts for lunch every single day to lose weight. Eating healthy is not about dietary restrictions; it's about learning to love healthy foods. Here is a list of other healthy sides to be on the lookout for and to keep on hand:

- Oranges
- Bananas
- Apples
- Avocados
- Tomatoes
- Broccoli
- Squash
- Corn
- Peas
- Grean Beans
- Sweet potatoes
- Carrots of any style
- Roasted veggies
- Grilled veggies
- Steamed veggies
- A garden salad with a light amount of dressing
- Baked Beans – These particular beans can be high in sugar, but beans are so crazy good for you that I think the sugar content is okay here.
- Bean salad
- Almonds
- Pistachios
- Walnuts
- Peanuts

This is a short list of foods to be sure to keep on hand, but any one of them makes for a healthy addition to your meal. I eat several of these foods, but just a few of them are needed to make real progress!

What worked for me

While I was on my weight loss journey I had to consistently make good choices and add a healthy food to my plate. I knew that my best chance of success would be to become more familiar with healthy foods and to eat something healthy for every meal. I had to *take action* by purposely trying new kinds of fruits and vegetables. Before long I started to crave squash and broccoli!

Here are some examples of how I accomplished this tactic:

1. I added baked beans and wheat buns to my favorite beef hot dogs.

2. Pizza was much better for me when I added a side salad (and ate less pizza).

3. When I ate chili I added corn bread to make a delicious meal.

4. Burgers were just as good with a sweet potato on the side instead of french fries.

5. Adding veggies to chicken and rice make the meal go much further, and there was no reason to feel guilty when getting a second helping!

6. Yellow squash could be added to just about anything, and was especially tasty in pasta meals.

Adding healthy choices to your meals isn't super complicated. Over time, this tactic gives you the chance to try many different healthy foods, and your body will begin to crave them. Once you get used to eating them and feeling the power of eating healthy, your body will start to fight back, and will begin to yearn for succulent veggies and fruits!

This Tactic Won't Work If I Go Out, Right?

My answer to this question is: not necessarily. Yes, going out to eat will often end up filling you with calories, extra fat, sodium, grease, and other crap. But adding a healthy side or a salad is still a good way to counteract this somewhat.

Instead of giving in completely, order a grilled chicken salad for dinner. That way, you can gorge yourself on dessert and not fret that you totally ruined your day.

Try to limit going out to eat, but when you really want to go out for a nice meal don't fret about it! Make better choices consistently, and continue pushing every day. The day you stop trying is the day you'll gain weight, get fat, and veer toward unhappiness. If you don't change your choices, the weight loss game will continue for the rest of your life.

If you do decide to make healthier choices, one bad day will not be the deciding factor in your success or failure. Keep pushing and keep making the best choices that you can and you'll succeed in the end.

Final Thoughts

This tactic is simple to try, just like the others. Give it a chance. The worst that can happen is you make a food you don't like and end up throwing it away or giving it away to a friend. No harm no foul, as you can always try something else at your next meal!

With these newfound powers of healthy eating the Fiber Guardian is more powerful than any foe. No cake monster nor brownie baker can stop him now. The Keebler Elf throws cookies at him, but with the unwavering power of his very own tactics, he smashes all but one cookie away.

With a mighty stalk of broccoli in his upraised hand he looks into the distance. His jaw drops and his vegetable weapon slides out of his hand and onto the ground below. A great and powerful foe has stepped out and is ready to do battle with the Fiber Guardian...

Tactic #9: Reduce Added Sugar Intake

My diet during college was craptastic. Yes, CRAPTASTIC! I ate way too much sugar and didn't even realize it. Between the overwhelming amount of sweets that I ate and the soda I imbibed daily, it's no wonder that I gained over 40 pounds.

Added sugar is the #1 thing to avoid if possible! However, don't let this warning deter you from eating fruits that are high in sugar. Natural sugars are okay and even encouraged, as the types of foods that contain it are necessary for a healthy diet.

What is the difference between natural sugars and added sugars? in brief, added sugars are found in cookies, cakes, ice cream, soda, candy, and other baked or processed foods. These foods are digested quickly with almost zero nutritional value.

Natural sugars found in milk and fruit bring with them precious vitamins and minerals and especially (you guessed it) fiber! The fiber in fruit helps the food to be digested more slowly and the spikes in blood sugar are not as dramatic as a result.

When I first decided to change my ways and eat healthier I limited my soda intake to the weekends. This wasn't the very best decision I could have made, but at the time it reduced my soda intake by over 50%! The key is to take small steps and do only what you're capable of doing.

Right now, I have made the commitment to be completely soda free, and my body thanks me for this decision. As I learned, the fastest route to your end goal is to start somewhere and head in the right direction!

Why You Should Avoid Added Sugars

Added sugar is pretty terrible for you across the board. It's associated with the cause of many diseases including:

- Type 2 diabetes, a disease that's a direct result of a diet that is too high in sugar. The body becomes resistant to insulin and this eventually leads to obesity.

- Obesity. Once the body becomes resistant to insulin it becomes harder to process foods with added sugars. This leads to an exponential effect on weight gain.

- Sugar is addictive! Dopamine is released upon eating sugar, which causes you to want more and more of whatever it is you just ate to give you that feeling!

- Too much sugar means that leptin resistance will occur. Leptin is a hormone in the brain that when released tells us to stop eating. However, too much sugar combats this due to its addictive nature. This just extrapolates the difficulty of losing weight!

- Sugar aids in the liver's ability to recover glycogen. However, most people who live sedentary lifestyles do not require their glycogen levels to be replenished. The liver turns excess sugar into fat instead!

To further illustrate this point, check out this infographic and article on what drinking just one can of coke can do to your body in just one hour (http://bit.ly/25oZOMr). It was enlightening to me, and certainly aided in my decision to stop drinking soda completely.

How to Reduce Added Sugars

While avoiding added sugar might seem daunting, it's definitely doable. By focusing on reducing sugar in all areas the goal can be accomplished. Here are a few practical ways to begin:

1. Start by replacing your soft drinks with water or fruit smoothies (think natural sugar instead of added!).

2. Become more aware of how much sugar you're eating by paying attention to food labels.

3. DO NOT replace high sugar foods with low fat or "diet" sodas. There is no proof that they actually help with weight loss, and there are studies that show a link between diet drinks and depression. Here are several more reasons why you should look elsewhere when trying to reduce your added sugar intake: http://bit.ly/21LlTjA.

4. Avoid excess candy. Candy is amazing, and I love eating it. However, you're basically just pouring spoonfuls of sugar down your gullet, and it just isn't worth it. That being said, a few starburst, or a candy bar now and then is okay. I do not completely abstain from added sugars, and doing so isn't life or death. However, if you find that you cannot control yourself and one starburst turns into 35, you might need to consider getting rid of candy completely!

5. When all else fails, a glass of water can be your best friend. Turn to it often and use it as your secret weapon against any and all slip ups!

6. Study your own diet currently. Remove any high sugar foods and replace with an alternative.

   • Too much soda? Drink more water.

   • Too many candy bars? Replace with your favorite fruit.

   • Too much fast food? Make your food at home.

   • Too much sugar in your favorite cereal? Try oatmeal instead.

   • Love to eat Ritz Bits? Try flavored almonds instead.

   • Drink a lot of juice? Switch to lemon water or hot flavored tea with a touch of honey instead!

7. Analyze food labels and arm yourself with the knowledge of how to spot foods with added sugars.

Final Thoughts on Reducing Added Sugars

Limiting your added sugar intake can be a major struggle. If you're in a place in life in which you eat a lot of sugar, stopping will prove difficult due to sugar's addictive nature. This tactic is probably one of the hardest ones in this book to put into practice, as processed food companies want us to be addicted so they keep earning money! We have to fight back or to give in to the drug.

You must fight the addiction to sugar, and you must begin to recognize the danger in continuing on your current path. Obesity is right around the corner when battling sugar addiction, and it is not a pretty sight. Being overweight brings with it many health related issues including depression. I believe that it's NEVER too late to make a change and turn things around. Start battling today, and make a decision that lowers your daily sugar intake.

An enemy has been exposed. The Sugar Beast has stepped out onto the playing field. The Fiber Guardian does the first thing he can think of and chucks a banana at the monstrosity. The banana scores a hit and the Sugar Beast bellows in outrage. Not really understanding, yet not willing to lose his advantage, the Fiber Guardian throws an apple and then a coconut. The coconut drops harmlessly after five feet but the apple strikes home, lodging itself in the maw of the Sugar Beast. Candy canes and gummy worms fly every which way as the Sugar Beast explodes into a shower of goodies. Covered from head to toe with sticky pieces of candy, but smiling proudly, the Fiber Guardian strides forward to face his next challenge.

Tactic #10: Increase Protein Intake

Protein is not just for those that want to bulk up and get huge. Protein is essential for anyone that is looking to lose weight. My basic understanding of protein used to be that you need extra protein to get bigger muscles. While this isn't necessarily false, protein is much more than that. Indeed, protein helps you to feel fuller for longer, acting much like fiber as it slows down your digestion.

Additionally, in one study, overweight women who increased protein intake from 15% to 30% of calories consumed 441 fewer calories per day. That's a huge caloric difference that would add up quickly. In fact, that's a 13,000 calorie difference per month, just by eating more protein!

When I was losing weight, I knew none of this. All I knew was that my focus was going to be on getting more fiber into my diet. I was going to be eating more high fiber foods if it killed me. I hardly even focused on protein.

But therein lies the beauty of the fiber/protein relationship. Fiber-rich foods are often rich in protein as well. When I was eating chili to have my fill of fiber for the day, I was getting an abundance of protein as well!

This was part of what worked so well for me, and part of why I think that the high-fiber diet is the way to go. But for this tactic, the focus is on protein, and I aim to convince you that eating more protein is a tactic you do not want to ignore.

Why should I eat more protein?

Here are several reasons why eating more protein is the way to go:

- As I mentioned above, eating more protein helps you to feel fuller for longer. This is because of a certain hormone that protein increases (peptide YY). This hormone specifically reduces appetite, which is obviously helpful when losing weight.

- Protein increases muscle mass which is the most well-known effect of eating protein. It's important to consider that increasing protein intake while on a diet will reduce the amount of muscle that is being broken down during the weight loss process. You'll lose more fat and less muscle if your protein intake is high.

- One study (http://1.usa.gov/1RkXn7C) claims that eating more protein is good for bone health, despite the common myth that it's not.

- Long-term weight loss can be achieved when protein is added to the diet as a common daily fixture. Making protein a priority will help you to achieve your weight loss goals, and will also aid in keeping the pounds off for good.

- Protein has been found to lower blood pressure. High blood pressure is one of the causes of stroke, heart attacks, and kidney disease, and eating more protein will reduce your chances of having any of these issues.

As I stated earlier, I started eating protein knowing only one of these facts. I ate it because I figured it would be a good idea to increase my protein intake with my lifting routine, and because I was already eating high fiber/ high protein foods and didn't even really need to think about it!

However, if you really want to up your protein intake right away, follow some of these tips below.

How to Eat More Protein

Increasing protein intake can seem like a daunting task, especially at first. Questions such as "What foods have protein?" and "How do I add these foods into my diet?" might flood your thoughts. However, it's less complicated than you think.

Keep in mind these simple steps in order to increase your protein intake and enjoy all of the associated health benefits.

1. Avoid crappy foods. I know, real scientific right? Be honest for a second, you KNOW what foods are bad for you. While some crappy foods have some protein (and I'm talking about REALLY bad foods), oftentimes they do not have any protein at all. Doritos, soda,

and any similar foods pack in calories through sugar and fat, without any added benefits.

2. Replace unhealthy foods with better, high-protein alternatives such as beans, broccoli, almonds, and meat such as chicken or fish.

3. Make a smoothie at home using a blender. Use Greek Yogurt to make the smoothie extremely high in protein, and add fruits to make it high in fiber.

4. Add a protein supplement to your homemade smoothies in order to get even more protein.

5. Men need to aim for about 56 grams of protein, and women need to aim for 46. This doesn't mean that you need to get EXACTLY this amount each day, but it's the average number to shoot for.

6. Slowly start adding more high protein foods into your diet and you'll be on the right track for sure!

That's all there is to it. It might seem a little difficult at first to incorporate high protein foods into your diet, but it's doable in time. Just keep making those small changes. Keep on adding these tactics into your weight loss repertoire for ultimate victory.

The war on weight loss was raging on for the Fiber Guardian. The Muffin Man and the Dorito Dork were giving him a run for his money and he felt himself slipping away. But yet… Off in the distance… a new hero appeared. A new hero to aid the Fiber Guardian in his quest. The Protein Kapow would bring balance to the force and together with the Fiber Guardian would ward off the onslaught of attacks from the enemy.

Tactic #11: Always Have Frozen Fruits and Vegetables Readily Available

Packing the fridge with healthy food was a major benefiting factor in my weight loss journey. I made sure that my freezer was packed with fruits and vegetables so that I'd always be able to throw blueberries into my smoothies, steam some broccoli, or add some carrots to a salad or stew.

The best way to lose weight and keep it off is to win battles in advance. Instead of keeping dessert constantly at your fingertips, keep your freezer packed with fruits and vegetables to always have healthy food readily available.

Worried about the quality of frozen fruits and veggies?

Good news! Frozen fruit and veggies are just as healthy (if not more healthy) than their fresh counterparts.

The Benefits of Frozen Produce

- Fresh fruits/veggies are picked before fully ripening and then sent to store shelves, enduring multiple temperature swings that decreases the freshness and nutritional value of the food. Studies by IFR Extra have shown that "fresh" produce can actually lose up to 45% of its beneficial nutrients during the time between being picked and being on your table, a potential time period of 16 days or more.

- Frozen fruits and veggies are picked when ripe, flash frozen, and then shipped in their frozen state. This method keeps the nutrients intact and the produce ready for you to snack on at peak quality. Fresh produce loses nutrients quickly, and frozen produce keeps for much longer.

- Beyond the nutritional difference between fresh and frozen, frozen produce is much more convenient. In the world of making weight loss easy, convenience is what we are going for here, as the journey is already difficult enough!

- Having frozen produce aids in fulfilling tactic #6 (Making dinner at home) and tactic #8 (eating something healthy for every meal) as it makes it even easier for you to make homemade masterpieces or even boring meals with a healthy side. (See below for links to recipes for awesome fruit and veggie meals!)

- It makes it easier for you because you do not necessarily have to plan ahead. All you need to do is acquire a bunch of frozen produce that you like and use it when you need it. Fresh produce might not last long enough for you to work it into your meals, and the pressure will be off of you to fit them in before they go bad!

That being said, it's true that nothing beats the taste of a fresh blueberry picked off the vine. If you find yourself near a farm where you can pick your own produce or buy directly from the farmer, I would not even dare tell you to buy frozen instead. Keep in mind that you can still go home and freeze it right away for use later on.

However, most people don't have this luxury, and the fresh fruit/veggies you'll find at grocery stores may not be as fresh as you might think.

Just about any way you look at it, going for frozen produce is the way to go. It will give you the ammunition you need to crush your weight loss goals.

Which Frozen Fruits and Veggies Should I Start With?

When you're shopping for fruits and veggies you can start by looking for the items listed below. This is by no means an exhaustive list, but it will give you a place to start!

Feel free to remove any of these from the list if you find that you don't like them, but it might be worth your while to give them a few chances. Also note that not all of these recipes are the healthiest recipes in the world. However, I believe that it's worth it to try the recipe as it introduces you to the flavor of that specific produce! A pineapple burger is worth the calories if it turns you on to pineapples. It's amazing what you can do with food, and the potential is great for you to find a meal that you love.

For each food type I've linked to a recipe (not my own) that would be a great way to test the waters, and find out if that type of produce is right for you.

1. Blueberries – Chicken & Blueberry Pasta Salad
   • http://bit.ly/1WPpTOI

2. Strawberries – Tuxedo Strawberries and Berry Crostini
   • http://bit.ly/1VNHw3e

3. Raspberries – Raspberry Oatmeal Cookies
   • http://bit.ly/1Scd65a

4. Kiwi – Strawberry Kiwi Smoothie
   • http://bit.ly/1MHRnQO

5. Mangoes – Fresh Mango Salsa Recipe
   • http://bit.ly/1Tadi9R

6. Pineapples – Pineapple Teriyaki Burgers
   • http://bit.ly/1MqKlVG

7. Cherries – Chocolate-Covered Cherry Baked Oatmeal
   • http://bit.ly/1RrfEMZ

8. Corn – Simple Summer Corn Soup
   • http://bit.ly/1WPq2Sh

9. Broccoli – Crispy Broccoli with Lemon and Garlic
   • http://bit.ly/1ZC7BT2

10. Carrots – Rosemary Roasted Carrots
    • http://bit.ly/1MqKsR8

11. Peas – Kheema Indian Spiced Ground Meat with Peas
    • http://bit.ly/1RsTYCg

12. Spinach – Spinach and Sun-Dried Tomato Stuffed Mushrooms
    • http://bit.ly/1UqOMmF

These foods will give you a starting point for what to have in your fridge. Continue reading for even more recipes tailored specifically to vegetables, and then fruits.

Easy Vegetable Meals

Here are a few meals you can make with frozen vegetables. I have simply taken the searching out of your hands, and compiled a list of great recipes for you. I didn't create these recipes, nor do I take credit for them. My aim is to give you the reader a direct link to some easy recipes to keep on hand for when you might need it.

- Brussels Sprouts with Lemon and Brown Rice
  - http://bit.ly/1ZC7HKe
- Sauteed Kale and Quinoa Skillet
  - http://bit.ly/1MHRxHM
- Oven-Roasted Potatoes and Vegetables
  - http://bit.ly/1RBI7yQ
- Teriyaki Veggie Bowls
  - http://bit.ly/1REw75T
- Crock Pot Vegetable Soup
  - http://bit.ly/1TaduG6

Easy Meals to Make Using Fruits

Fruit's an amazing and delicious food. It often lasts longer than vegetables, and it's not always necessary to freeze it. Apples can last quite a while in the fridge, and bananas don't freeze well (unless you cut them up first). However, berries, pineapple slices, mangos, and other tropical fruit freeze well, and make for great additions to many different types of meals.

Here are some of those meals. Again, I'm not claiming credit for the below mentioned recipes, I'm merely suggesting these links as a good resource for you to make some awesome meals with your frozen fruits.

- Greek Yogurt Fruit Tart
  - http://bit.ly/1Sm8lss
- Mojito Fruit Salad
  - http://bit.ly/1WPqcZV
- Light and Healthy Fruit Dip
  - http://bit.ly/1RsUaS3
- Frozen Fruit Yogurt Bites
  - http://bit.ly/1TadztA
- Raspberry Zinger Energy Balls
  - http://bit.ly/1WPqct7

Well there you have it! Plenty of awesome recipes to start using right away. Go out and get yourself some frozen produce, and you'll find that eating healthy can be quite an enjoyable experience.

Tactic #12: Occasionally Eat the Treats You Love

Occasional indulgence is one of the keys to losing weight, especially at first. You might not hear that very often from other weight loss experts, but I'm not like those other experts. I'm just like any one of you. I'm merely stating what worked for me, because it WORKED FOR ME. If it worked for me, it could work for you too, don't you think?

I knew that if I wanted to lose weight, I had to enjoy the process and make changes slowly. I eventually quit soda altogether, but doing so took time. I was not able to quit soda cold turkey, especially when I had been drinking soda almost every day.

Your level of commitment and pace of change might be different than my own. I was a 23 year old kid who could stand to take it slow. I recognize that some of you readers might be older, and that is perfectly okay. You might be under the direction of your doctor to make some MASSIVE changes right away.

However, this doesn't mean that you need to stop eating food that you love altogether. I believe that there is healthy and delicious food out there to meet anyone's needs. It just might take some time to find out what that food is, especially if you're determined to make massive changes right away.

For those of you that can afford to take your time, don't be afraid to eat a brownie or have a soda, as long as you don't let that decision get you down. Own the brownie, enjoy the soda, and continue to crush your goals.

Some Tips on Indulgence

Indulging on foods can be a good thing as it allows you to not have to quit cold turkey from a food, but it can also be a bad thing. Eating that brownie or having that can of soda could put you on the fast track to failure if you're not careful.

Here are some tips to keep in mind when deciding to indulge in your favorite foods.

- Recognize that you'll go overboard at times. When I first started my high-fiber diet, I would eat high-fiber foods during the week, but then Friday came. I would eat a Steak stromboli with fries and a big bottle of Mountain Dew to reward myself. This worked in that I was able to lose weight, but my system let me have it; Saturday was a rough day on my insides!

- Remember that we're all human. Even if we're doing really well, there will be times that we make poor dietary decisions. Luckily for you I wrote a blog post that covers how to <u>recover from a lousy dietary decision</u>.

- Limit the indulgence to one dessert, or a certain drink with a normal meal. The less you shock your system the better. It's best not to have a full "cheat day" and instead spread out that indulgence with a cheat here or there through the week. This becomes easier over time, as your body adjusts to eating healthier foods and you notice a huge difference in how you feel when you aren't depriving your body of those precious nutrients.

- Plan ahead for the indulgence. Plan for a piece of chocolate cake for dessert after dinner. This way you'll be prepared for it, and you can even look forward to it. Knowing that Friday's meal will consist of a delicious dessert can help you press forward and make positive choices all week.

- Stay hydrated! Never underestimate the power of drinking water.

I found that indulging every once in awhile was extremely helpful in my weight loss journey. I was able to look forward to eating the "good" foods, and that helped me to limit my intake of bad foods during the week. It was a great way for me to start.

Figure out what your weight-loss goals are, and decide for yourself if this tactic might be helpful. Some people should probably try to quit cold turkey and avoid certain foods forever if they can't control their intake.

Remember to stay hydrated, plan ahead, place limits on yourself, and to not beat yourself up if you overindulge. None of us are perfect and we're bound to make mistakes from time to time.

Stay on track, and eventually the small changes will add up to victory!

Oops! The Fiber Guardian was caught with his hands in the cookie jar... Again! The Keebler Elf cackles as FG falls to his knees, crying "Nooo!" As he stares at the ground, he remembers the taste of apples and whole wheat pasta. He clenches his hands into fists, and rises. With a resolute expression FG stares at the elf and says "You can't get me down little man, tomorrow is a brand spanking new day." The Fiber Guardian smiles as he offers the pouting elf a carrot, and rests peacefully knowing that cookies will not spell his downfall.

Tactic #13: Bring Healthy Snacks to Work

The workplace can be a major derailer of weight loss programs. The temptations are all too real and constant. We don't live in a society that promotes healthy eating and decisions. We live in a society where obesity is accepted and overweight people live in a resigned acceptance of their bodies.

It doesn't need to be this way.

When I worked as a mobile therapist I spent a lot of time in the car between clients. I was constantly driving by fast food places every block. It was hard not to stop and grab a quick bite to eat, especially if I had brought nothing with me that day.

When I was promoted and worked in an office setting, things got even worse. There was ALWAYS junk food in the office. From donuts during meetings, to candy jars full of chocolate, it was easy to get carried away and have a terrible day. To make matters even worse, you're stuck in the office all day, with nothing to burn off those calories except the walk to the water cooler or the bathroom, or the daily wrestle with the copy machine.

Where I work now, I'm thankfully moving around all day. I don't have to worry about spending the day being sedentary as I'm constantly up and doing physical labor. Working in a retirement home has been awesome, but the food temptations can be even worse, as I work through all of the meals each day! I literally have to say "no" if I do not want dessert when our servers take our orders. It's hard to constantly say no to pumpkin pie and chocolate cake.

Regardless of where you work or what kind of work you do, bringing your own snacks into work can be a major boon for your weight loss goals.

Foods to Bring to Work

The best foods to bring to work include ones that are easily stored in a small container or fridge. If you have your own office or fridge, the types of food you can choose from is unlimited. However, if you have a mobile job and work out of your car, chances are you don't have the luxury of a fridge. To account for the snack-limiting jobs, this list will include foods that are easily accessible and easily stored.

- Staple fruits such as apples, bananas, and oranges should never be taken for granted. They are easily eaten and easily carried. Try your best to keep these foods within your reach!

- Other fruit such as pre-cut pineapple, kiwi, and mangoes can make for a delicious and refreshing afternoon snack.

- Any type of nut such as an almond, pistachio, cashew, or walnut. Nuts are small, yet they are packed with protein, fiber, and beneficial fats.

- Fiber bars (Nugo Fiber Bars, Kind Bars, Clif Bars, Etc.), or protein bars. Just try to avoid the bars that are high in sugar, and those that contain ANY trans fat! Most bars are not natural, and thus should not be heavily relied upon as your only source of food. However, compare just about any fiber bar to a Krispy Kreme donut and you would be hard pressed to argue that fiber bars are the worse decision here. A huge plus is that they are extremely convenient, and can be put just about anywhere.

- Try putting carrots and celery in a baggie with a little bit of ranch dip on the side. This is a MUCH healthier snack than a bag of chips. and only takes a little bit of time to put together.

- Greek Yogurt

- Homemade Granola

- Homemade popcorn. Yes, popcorn is indeed good for you as it's high in fiber!

- Hard boiled eggs

- String cheese

- Unsweetened dried fruit such as raisins or cranberries.

- For more ideas check out these Healthy Snack Ideas for Busy People: http://bit.ly/1pCl2FN.

The next time you think about stopping for a quick "bite" to eat at your local Burger King, you'll be prepared to pull out a banana and a fiber bar from your bag instead! You will be much more nourished, and feel way more satisfied than any thousand calorie fast food burger would make you feel.

Bringing your own healthy snacks gives you the ammunition you need to say no when offered other food at the office. It helps you to avoid the cravings fast food can bring on by giving you the option to fill up on power food instead of high fat, high salt, high sugar, and poor choices.

Work can be a tough place to keep up with your weight loss goals. With this tactic in your back pocket, you'll start to win battles and you'll start to see results!

Tactic #14: Have Another Cup of Jo

If you're one of the 83% of adult Americans that drink coffee every single day, then you're probably excited to read about this tactic. Indeed, when used in moderation and combined with other weight loss tactics, coffee drinking can be a nice addition to your strategy. Drinking more coffee can actually be a great way to lose weight, as it speeds up our metabolism by causing thermogenesis which is our body's way of creating heat when metabolizing food.

I started to drink coffee when I was trying to lose weight. I was always told that I would eventually drink coffee, and I would learn to savor its taste. Of course, I never believed anyone that told me this, but I was wrong!

Coffee became a part of my daily routine. I would drink it every morning with a donut from the local gas station. The donut eventually became a cereal bar, which then became a fiber bar during the later stages of my weight loss journey. But coffee was there, right in the thick of it all, just waiting for me to drink it each and every day. Of course, I happily obliged, and little did I know that it was doing a great thing by furthering my weight loss efforts.

The Truth about Coffee Drinking for Weight Loss

The hard truth is that coffee alone will not solve all of your weight problems. You cannot expect that just because you're drinking coffee, the weight will just start to come off. It won't work that way. If you add just one coffee a day to your diet, you might see a small difference, but it won't do much if you spend every day eating pizza and lounging in front of the TV.

There are several reasons why coffee can help you to lose weight.

Why Drinking Coffee Helps you to Lose Weight

1. The caffeine in coffee increases your body's metabolism and facilitates the burning of body fat.

2. Coffee decreases your appetite by helping you to feel more full.

3. Having a cup of coffee before a workout gives you more energy and will help you to get the most out of your workout. Coffee is also a powerful antioxidant, which is important for post-workout recovery. I usually have a cup of coffee before a workout, and I find that my workouts go much better because of this!

4. Coffee is devoid of its own calories, so it makes for a good low-calorie drink to have with a meal.

5. To a lot of people coffee tastes great. Having something you can look forward to and that you know is going to taste awesome is a good part of the process of losing weight.

Now that you know how coffee can help you to lose weight, you're probably ready to go and grab yourself a cup. Before you do that, check out the next part for tips to remember when drinking coffee.

Tips on Coffee Drinking for Weight Loss

- Don't overdo it. It can be dangerous to have too much caffeine. Drink no more than 3-5 cups (8oz per cup) per day. (A Starbucks tall is 12oz, a grande 16oz, a venti 24oz, and a trenta 31oz.) If you find yourself getting too much, try weaning off of coffee for a short period. It only takes about 5 days for your body's receptor cells to refresh, meaning that your first cup when you come back will feel like a million bucks!

- Avoid too much cream and sugar. When I first started drinking coffee I used a lot of cream and a lot of sugar. Nowadays, I only use a small amount of creamer and no sugar. Drinking it black would obviously be the best way to do it, but I'm not to that point yet. My wife drinks it black, and I can with some coffee flavors, but I need a little bit of cream in most cases.

- Pace yourself throughout the day. Don't have an extra large cup of jo in the morning, and then nothing throughout the rest of the day. This is usually too much too soon. Right around 2 o'clock you'll start to feel drowsy and will either need to reach for another cup of coffee, take a nap, or just deal with it. I usually have one cup of coffee in the morning, and one or two in the afternoon. That way I"m not overdoing it.

- Try some bulletproof coffee. You mix the bulletproof coffee brand with unsalted butter for a creamy and healthy coffee. It's supposedly very good for you!

All in all, starting out your day with a cup of coffee (and water of course!) is one of the best things you can do to meet your goals. If you love coffee as much as I do, take heart that drinking it can be helpful! Just remember the tips I shared, and you'll start to see results.

As the fight continued a secret weapon appeared on the battlefield. It was one the enemy mistook for aid in their cause, but how wrong they were. Coffee, oh wonderful and amazing coffee, was on the Fiber Guardian's side. The splendor of the caffeine filled superdrink would fill him with power and would speed his footsteps. The end goal of defeating Lackadaisical loomed ever closer.

Section 3

GETTING PHYSICAL WITH WEIGHT LOSS

Living an active lifestyle is not hard once you get going. It actually can be a lot of fun! I think that being active throughout my life has always helped me, and I will forever appreciate my parents for teaching me tennis, and pushing me to play outside!

It might take time to get used to if you're used to sitting in an office all day proceeded by driving home and lounging on the couch. It isn't easy to change from this low level of activity, but it's possible. Through the tactics that I will share here, you can start to live a much more active lifestyle by making slow and positive changes.

Once you start becoming active and once you start to get used to doing more active things you'll start to crave the chance to get outside and run, play a game of tennis, or to go swimming in the pool. Trust me, that might seem like a joke to you, but it isn't. Once you start to enjoy the feelings associated with a workout when those endorphins are released, you'll want to start doing things every day!

The tactics I'm going to share here might be obvious to some of you. They might also be ones you've tried before with little success. As with the tactics that I shared with eating, not all of them will help you, but my aim is to give you plenty of tools to fill your weight-loss superhero toolkit. I will also share how it worked for me when I implemented these strategies during my weight loss journey. You'll see that it's possible to lose weight and have fun doing it!

Tactic #15: Find Something Active That You Love to do

When I was growing up I played tennis constantly. My dad, brother, and I would go out 3-4 times per week and hit around the ol ball of... hmm, what is a tennis ball made of? Anyway. We would go out and play often. It was an awesome time to hang out with family, but it was also a great workout as we really pushed each other to do our absolute best.

And the best part? It didn't feel like a boring workout! We were not going to the courts to just lose a few pounds, we were going to have fun. Man! What a difference that can make! I think this is probably why so many workouts like Zumba, Insanity, and Crossfit have become popular; they are so much fun to do. Having fun, getting a good workout, and spending time with my family all at the same time was an excellent way for me to spend my time.

After college it took some time for me to figure out what to do that was a good activity. I spent a lot of time going to the gym because I wasn't sure what else to get into! Eventually, I joined my church's softball team, and my wife and I played ultimate frisbee in a league. I was motivated to go to the gym in between times to supplement my weight loss goals, as well as become stronger and be more competitive in the leagues I was in because of course, the Fiber Guardian wanted to triumph and do the best that he could do.

My first year of softball was a challenge because I was still pretty chunky from college. It wasn't until my second season until I started to run faster, hit harder, and play the field better. Most everyone commented on my weight loss, and it definitely showed in my ability to play the game. This spurred me on to keep with it and to keep the weight off for good.

Today, my wife constantly says that she finds it so much easier to play a game of ultimate frisbee than to go for a short jog. I definitely agree with her on this. We play as much ultimate frisbee as we can. It's not only a great workout, but an excellent way for us to spend time together. We love playing, and we love the rush of playing together on a team. It has helped us both to stay in shape and to have something that we are working towards continuously.

It has definitely been a journey to figure out how to stay active and not become bored with exercise. Going to the gym every single day was hard for me, and can be hard for a lot of people. It just isn't exciting enough to keep me interested for a long period of time. I have found that you truly need to find something that you love in order to have fun and lose weight consistently.

If you don't enjoy the exercise you get, you'll stop making an effort and lose all the progress you've made. And it will only get harder to start next time. Don't fall into the cycle that millions of dieters do: starting and stopping diets and exercise programs, only to find themselves more overweight than when they started. The Action Diet is a lifestyle change and is one that you can do on a consistent basis.

With that being said, and because I believe sincerely in the power of finding an active hobby that will motivate and push you to reach your goals, I have compiled a list of some awesome hobbies that you can try out. The idea isn't to do all of these things, but to find a few that you just love to do! Find a sport or game that invigorates your soul; join a league; make a new friend; WHATEVER you can do to be active, do it. Make it happen, superheroes!

A Big List of Fun and Active Hobbies

Pick one or two of the following activities and get to it. Already do some of these? Well, you're way ahead of most, but answer me this – how often do you do that activity? Chances are that the answer is not enough. Get out there, enjoy yourself, and start making some progress.

Here are just some of the activities you could begin to enjoy right away. This list is not exhaustive by any means, but these activities will get you headed in the right direction:

- Walking – Start walking everywhere that you can! Walking can be a lot of fun, especially if you're into audiobooks like I am. I love to take a stroll and listen to a good book, especially when the weather is nice.

- Tennis – Tennis is a lifelong sport that only takes a court, a few balls, a racket, and a friend.

- Racquetball – Sets can be found at a lot of gyms, and it's a great workout.

- Ping Pong – Ping Pong may not seem like much, but if you get into it, you'll find yourself sweating soon shortly into playing.

- Volleyball – It's a great team sport for having fun. Do 2v2 or 3v3 for the best physical impact.

- Swimming – Swimming is one of the best exercises for you, because you don't put as much stress on your joints as you do when running on pavement or lifting weights.

- Ultimate Frisbee – My personal favorite sport ever. It's very similar to soccer in that you spend most of your time running. It's also one of the best sports for burning calories!

- Disc golf – It's not as intense as ultimate frisbee, but you do get a lot of walking in when playing this sport.

- Hiking – Hiking is a great way to enjoy nature and get a workout in all at the same time

- Surfing – I have never surfed, but if you're near a beach, why not try this out?

- Parkour – I would be too scared of breaking my ankles, but doing parkour or freerunning is a great way to stay active.

- Dancing – Just dancing around the house is good enough for this one, but you can indeed get into dance as a hobby too!

- Gardening – Yes gardening is a great hobby to get into and a great way to shed off some extra pounds.

- Kickball – I think kickball is super boring actually, but I have a lot of friends that love it for some reason that I will never understand. But that's just my opinion. Don't knock it until you try it!

- Any league sport, such as soccer, flag football, or basketball.

- Biking

- Softball or baseball

- Boxing
- Weight lifting
- Running

Just find something that you enjoy. We were created to be active people, not people that sit around and watch TV all day!

The Benefits of Getting Involved in Something Active

Finding an activity that you love to do can make all the difference in the world for you, and not just for the workout you get by going to these places. There are many benefits that finding an activity can do for you. These benefits include:

1. When the competition rises, your level of commitment will rise too. Whether you're on a volleyball team, a rising squash star, or a wakeboarding champion, the urge to get better at the activity will drive you to new heights. Personally, I strive to get better at ultimate frisbee, and I know that every time I'm working out at the gym it helps me to get better at ultimate. Every time I take the field I give 110% in order to reach my highest potential. The more you enjoy the activity, the more you'll feel the urge to master it!

2. Community. Being involved in an activity with other people helps us to feel like we belong. We all strive to be a part of something, and a sense of community is a strong motivator to keep on moving forward and making gains. It's harder to say "no!" to working out when the workout for the day is the championship volleyball game.

3. Consistency. When you join a league or get into a hobby that you love, you'll be doing that activity consistently. Rome wasn't built in a day, and so too you need to find something that you're doing consistently in order to see long-term change. This tactic can be perfect for you as it will help you to look forward to being active on a regular basis.

4. You will have fun. Having fun is paramount to losing weight and being healthy. It's much much harder to lose weight if you're just going through the motions and dreading each workout. The gym can be a fun place for some, but if it isn't a place you look forward

to going to, then it isn't going to do a lot of good for you in the long run! Just like we can't eat carrots and apples all day because we would get bored of it, so too we cannot begrudgingly go through the motions of working out. We need to enjoy life to truly make a change!

In the end, the core benefit of being active is to lose weight and become more healthy. Every single one of us would be lying if we didn't have that goal for ourselves. We all want to reach our goals, even if that desire is deep within us, hidden by the cobwebs of shame, regret, or the fear of failure. Find something active that you love to do and do it, and you'll see results. You will start to be able to push back those nasty cobwebs and you'll find happiness.

A frisbee came flying out of nowhere and was caught by the Fiber Guardian. FG instantly felt a surge of power flow through his veins. With a deep huck of the disc he leveled up to warrior status. As he ran his smile widened. The stars themselves would be jealous of the shine on his face as he reveled in newly discovered truth; no enemies were near. Not even Lackadaisical, the wizard of restless endeavors, could enter the hallowed ground of this grassy arena.

Tactic 16: Walk Everywhere That You Can

Walking is so easy, a caveman did it. Walking has been done since the beginning of creation. The first people didn't drive, nor did they ride in fancy motorcycles. The only form of public transportation would have been a small tribe walking together. Walking is the original form of travel.

Walking is even one of the first major events in our life. For many of us, the event is celebrated by our entire family as our first foray into becoming a full blown toddler. As children we walk, run, skip, climb, dance, and otherwise enjoy moving our bodies in all kinds of ways. This is one reason why most kids don't have problems keeping weight off, because they are way more active than most parents can keep up with. Kids *want* to move around and love to play.

However, unless this is encouraged by parents, this level of activity will start to wane much faster than it was intended. A teenager burdened with homework is not going to be as energetic as a child, and an adult burdened with adulthood is not nearly as energetic as a teenager. This is the natural progression of things. But if we don't stay active, weight loss problems will ensue.

Childhood obesity is one of the saddest preventable "disease" outbreaks in American history. It's caused by a great many factors, but I believe it could be eradicated with an upbringing focused on the importance of staying active and making healthy food choices. Parents: your kids are MUCH better off if you raise them from the beginning with a healthy lifestyle. Just start by walking with them when they are young and continue walking as they get older. It will benefit you personally, but you'll also see the positive effects that your guidance will have on the lives of your children. Just keep walking, just keep walking...

Walking is one of easiest forms of exercise and yet it's one of the most underrated as well. According to an article on Prevention.com walking is healthier than running (http://bit.ly/1Rrg5H6). It proposes that running over long periods is stressful on your body and can cause damage in the long run. The article does cite several studies that it claims backs up its conclusions.

I advise you to check out the article and formulate your own opinion on the matter. I would not go as far as to say that you should replace running completely with walking, especially if you love to run, but I would say that walking might be a lot better for you than you might realize. It's the most underrated and underutilized weight loss tool available to you. It's much easier on your body for sure, and you don't need to be highly trained to do it. It's easy to do it consistently, as your body will not get too sore from walking, even if you choose to walk several miles.

Initializing a walking routine is a no brainer and is a solid tactic for weight loss.

My Walking Story

I started walking consistently with my wife soon after we got married. It became routine for us to go on certain loops around the neighborhood just to breathe in the fresh air. Neither of us were doing it to up our level of fitness. We were just doing it to spend time together outside and enjoy life together. Little did I know that walking was one of the best things I could be doing for my health.

Over time we started creating longer walking loops and I found that walking was one of my favorite activities. We eventually walked a loop of 4 miles pretty consistently, and it didn't even seem like it was that long. We loved to spend an hour or more walking and found that our moods always improved by the end.

Not only did I get to spend quality time with my best friend, but I got to discuss life, brainstorm for the future, and lose weight all at the same time. It was on a walk that we decided that we wanted more than to just stay with our current jobs. It was walking that got the ideas flowing about moving out of state, and it was walking that bridged our connection with God and our prayers were answered. We spent countless walks praying that our move would become a reality and that we would no longer feel stuck in our current place.

Walking allowed our minds to escape the confines of feeling trapped that we felt at our apartment and our jobs, and it allowed us to see more clearly that our potential was much more than we were currently achieving.

This simple act of putting one foot in front of the other changed my life. If you want to change your own life I suggest you sneaker up, get off the couch, and walk!

Reasons to Walk

There are countless reasons why walking is a great idea. Here are ten of the most powerful reasons you should treat this tactic like weight-loss gold.

1. Walking after meals lowers blood pressure – Walking is one of the easiest ways to tackle high blood pressure. If you take to walking, especially after meals, you can lower your blood pressure by increasing your heart rate and strengthening your heart muscle.

   There are many other ways to lower blood pressure such as avoiding salty foods and reducing stress, but those who work in stressful environments and enjoy salty tastes might find these solutions too difficult. Walking, even at a slow pace, can be a perfect way to battle high blood pressure.

2. Walking can reduce the risk of some cancers – Reducing the risk of cancer is something that everyone would like to do for themselves. There is no one alive that isn't at least a tad bit fearful of hearing from their doctor, "You have cancer." To lessen the chances that this fear becomes a reality for you, start taking better care of yourself today. Getting into the habit of going for regular walks can reduce breast cancer by 25%, reduced risk of lung cancer, colon cancer, and bowel cancer.

3. Reduced risk of heart disease from walking – The results are in. Increasing your steps by just 2000 per day can decrease your risk of heart disease by over 10%! That's a staggering victory for the folks that decide to take a little jaunt around the neighborhood. With the average American only getting about 5000 steps per day (well under the recommended rate of 10,000 steps per day) all signs point to the need for us all to walk more.

4. Immune system performance is boosted – In a study that followed over 1000 men and women, walking at least 20 minutes a day proved to be enough to provide a significant boost to the immune system. Walking reduced the number of days sick by a whopping 43%!

    Think about that for a quick second. All it takes is *walking* around for a measly 20 minutes a day to boost your immune system and prevent illness. Wouldn't you rather be up and moving than sick in bed?

5. People who walk regularly live longer – Living a sedentary lifestyle could indeed kill you. Sitting in front of a TV for hours on end eating fast food will be sure to lead you down the wrong path. It doesn't have to be this way though! Walking is easy, and doing it could indeed help you to live a longer, more fulfilling life. Just walking 20 minutes a day is enough to reap the health benefits of walking!

6. Walking reduces stress levels – Walking is a great way to get out and shake off the stress of the day. I do this in my own life to digest the day, and to move on from things I cannot change. Walking, especially on a nice day, helps to relax the mind and soothe the soul.

    For more on this see How Does Exercise Reduce Stress from Everybody Walks.org. There are very interesting facts about stress that relate to walking that can be found in this article.

7. Creative synapses in the brain can be fired when walking outdoors, especially in younger children – Getting outside and walking, especially with a group, is a proven method of decreasing stress, and increasing positivity. Nothing beats the sights, sounds, and smells of a stroll down a nature path or a jaunt in the woods.

    Furthermore, walking in nature and spending time away from electronic devices improved the problem solving ability of the group (in the study linked to above) by a full 50%.

8. Walking allows our conscious mind to take in all that is around us – So often when inside staring at computer screen I start to feel my mind drifting away. Compared to the clar-

ity and mindfulness that I feel when I'm outdoors, it's a wonder why I ever choose to sit down in front of a screen!

There is even such a thing as walking meditation. Normally we think of meditation as sitting on the ground in a crossed legged position humming to ourselves. This does not always have to be the case, as meditation is more about mindfulness and being aware of what is going on around you.

9. Walking does not require any special equipment – One of the best parts about walking is that you don't need to spend a lot of money to get into it! Chances are you probably already have a good pair of shoes, and that is pretty much IT as far as equipment.

Depending on where you live, you might need to invest in some Under Armour or a heavy rain jacket, but you probably already own some sort of cold weather gear.

10. You can walk in any type of weather – For the most part bad weather is no excuse for not being able to go for a walk. Unless you have a physical handicap that might make it dangerous, walking in bad weather can be quite fun!

One of the earliest memories my wife and I have together is going for a walk at night in the **freezing rain**. It was probably dangerous, and we probably could have gotten hurt, but nothing bad happened. On the contrary, we had an absolute BLAST sliding down the end of this wooden bridge that spans the creek of our college alma mater. We talked about it constantly in the days following, and it comes up every once in awhile as a fond memory for us.

The point is, walking in any weather can lead to great experiences which create great memories. If we'd sat inside and watched a movie, I can guarantee you that we would not have remembered that night.

For even more reasons to walk, see this full page on my site: (http://bit.ly/21Lmxxq). It includes the above reasons to walk, with 15 more to learn about. (If you can't tell already I love walking.)

I even wrote this chapter after a 2.5 mile walk. I believe this shows that I do indeed walk the walk.

Where to Walk

Figuring out where to walk was a problem that I didn't have until very recently. I was always able to just take a stroll in my neighborhood and walk anywhere that I wanted to. But after moving to a small town in North Carolina I found out that not every neighborhood has sidewalks. This should have been obvious to me, but it truly shook up my routine. I live and work in one building off the beaten path. The only sidewalks in the area exist around the perimeter of my building. I can't safely walk to any major road, and I'm nowhere near any real place that I can go and write.

1. This presented many questions for my wife and me:

2. What would we do to work out?

3. How would we still walk?

How could we escape from work while we are off as we live on site?

At first we became pretty negative and were wondering if things would really work out. Were we destined to feel miserable and stuck, without even a place to walk?

We soon realized that no, of course we would not be stuck. We are both happy people, but we are also realizing even more that we are both highly adaptable people.

To combat our immediate need we found a local gym and joined up. We would walk on the treadmill if that was our only option. Then we found a family friend in a nearby town that was nice enough to let us use her home as a base from which we could walk from. The nearby town is full of sidewalks and soon became a second home for us. This allowed us to escape from work, take a walk, and get a solid workout in.

It didn't happen overnight, but we problem solved and figured out a way to overcome our obstacles. If you find yourself in the same boat, try some of the below strategies for finding a way to walk:

1. Join a gym and use a treadmill. It's not ideal or even that much fun, but it's an option.

2. Search for a local park.

3. Find a place to drive to, and then walk there. Even if it's 20-30 minutes away it's worth it to be able to get outside and walk around.

4. Take a step back, problem solve, and sort through your options. Regardless of your situation there has to be an answer, even if it isn't ideal.

Walking Tips

Here are some quick tips to remember when walking:

- Be sure to watch where you're going. I wouldn't tell you this if I didn't have to constantly remind myself as well. I have almost walked out into traffic several times when walking outside. Be careful so your walking journey doesn't end in tragedy.

- Use a Fitbit and track your steps. Not much is more satisfying than schooling all of your friends and family in the competitions because you went on a 5 mile walk.

- Try out Audible from Amazon. It's a great thing to pair with walking as you can listen to some great books and enjoy the outdoors at the same time.

- Walk with a friend or loved one. You will grow closer together, and the deep conversations you'll have will become more and more meaningful as you grow closer together.

Walking is one of the best tactics you have to begin losing weight. Try it now and enjoy the feeling of the great outdoors (or feeling of the gym if that is the route you go!)

BONUS: To help you get started with walking, I've created a PDF walking calendar. It will help you start walking every day, and will keep you accountable if you reference it throughout the month!

Get it right here: http://bit.ly/1WPqBeW.

Tactic #17: Train for a 5K

What!? You want me to actually run a 5k!? What are you, a crazy person!?

No I'm not crazy, and yes you can do it. I don't care if you actually run an official 5k race or not; that's up to you. While running a race is pretty exhilarating (and can be a crazy amount of fun, especially if you do a color run), I think that the prep work and the time spent training for the race is where you see most benefits. But if you're training for a race you might as well run the durned thing too.

Running the race will allow you to test your limits and to push yourself further than you would have ever realized possible. When you complete your first 5k, you'll realize that it was indeed possible for you. You can relish in the fact that you completed a 3.1 mile jaunt, and you can set your sights even higher!

I ran in a color run, and I didn't even train for it. I didn't do well. I had to take several breaks and wasn't able to run it straight through. I wish that I had trained for it, because I would have been able to run it straight through at a pretty good pace.

After the race, my wife and I ran more often than we ever had before. Seeing how we did compared to other people really pushed us to try to get better. We eventually got to the point where we would hit our stride and be able to run for miles straight without stopping.

I honestly never thought that I would be able to get to that point. I had never before run a mile straight, let alone 3.1 miles! I had always played sports that had running at intervals, not marathons. Ultimate frisbee was intense for sure, but I was always able to stop and rest for a bit, even just a few seconds of rest. After the race, it took a lot of training to be able to hit a pace and maintain that pace.

Running the race was well worth it, and it paid dividends in post-race motivation.

Why You Should Train for a 5K

Training for a 5K is all about setting a goal and working towards that goal. At times, the weight loss journey can be too connected to the numbers on the scale. When you set goals in addition to weight loss, the weight will come off as a by-product of reaching for other things.

When you find yourself running every day just so you can increase your pace, run further, and run longer, you'll find that the weight will start to come off! The best part is that the focus shifts from wanting to lose the weight to wanting to do the best you can in the race. This represents a monumental shift in thinking that leads to a lifestyle in which you're healthy, active, and loving life.

Training gives you the opportunity to reach your full potential. It gives you the chance to be the best you can be!

How to train for a 5K

Training for a 5K doesn't have to be a difficult process. It can be as simple as getting out there every day and pushing yourself harder with each run. In the time after the color run I didn't consult any official 5K running strategy. I just went out 3-4 times per week and ran. I eventually was able to run further each day.

I kept pushing myself until I was able to run a 5K without stopping. I was then able to run even farther at a continually faster pace. My tips for training for a 5K are pretty straight forward:

1. Go out and run 3-4 times per week.

2. Consistently do this for at least a month.

3. Push yourself as hard as you can to get better by running further and faster.

4. Don't be afraid to walk when you need to. Walk until you catch your breath and then run again.

5. Mix in at least one day of interval running to increase your speed.

6. Remember that you're going to have your really good days and your really bad days. Some days you'll feel like you can run forever, and some days you'll want to collapse after the first mile. Don't beat

yourself up; just get out there and do the best that you can. In the end that is all that you can do! Give 100%, recover, and keep at it.

See this article on Active.com for a more in depth look at how to train for a 5K: http://bit.ly/1pCli7N.

Running Tips

Some of these tips might seem obvious, but they were ones that I learned throughout my training period.

- Get a good pair of shoes.
- Stay hydrated with water or a few sips of gatorade (don't go overboard on the sugary drinks like this, but it can indeed be a good boost during a run or a good kickstart).
- Set a goal before each run and see how you do. This will serve to push you and for you to be able to see the progress you're making.
- Start each run with a walk or a really light jog to get the body ready.
- Only run at night if you have the proper equipment.
- Remember to run on the left side of the road facing traffic (US).
- Get enough sleep at night in order to properly recover from a long run or an intense workout.

Most of the time, you'll have to make some mistakes yourself and discover what works for you and your body. However, starting out with a little extra knowledge can help to avoid injury and losing interest early on.

Most importantly, remember that training is all about finding what works for you and pushing yourself. Be consistent, and before you know it you'll be running 5Ks with ease!

Tactic #18: Lifting for Weight Loss

Many people think of weight lifting solely as a means of "bulking up" or gaining weight. The common image that comes to mind is of a massive body builder with a small head who is grunting and throwing weights around in the gym. While that's the cliche, that meathead is not carrying around a lot of extra fat.

This is due to the fact that lifting weights is really good for losing weight. Strength training actually aids in burning more fat after the fact while your body is recovering from lifting. Adding in a few strength training sessions to your weekly exercise routine can make a world of difference in your weight loss goals!

Moreover, being sore from lifting makes you feel like you're getting somewhere and can be a boost psychologically in my opinion! Even though it might not feel great walking up the stairs the next day, pushing your body to the limit really makes you feel like you're going in the right direction, and this can make all the difference at times! I found this to be very true during my initial weight loss journey.

The fact of the matter is that lifting weights (or resistance training) can help you to become leaner, fit into the clothes you want to fit into, and ultimately really see the difference when you look into the mirror. You are able to realize the goal of looking sexy and being healthy without even having to worry about what the numbers on the scale say.

My Weight Lifting Story

Weight lifting was something I did off and on while in college. I would go for long stretches of lifting several times per week and then would lose interest and stop. This, in addition to a really poor diet, was not going to help me to lose weight. On the contrary, as you all know by now, I gained a lot of weight during my 4 year college stint.

It wasn't until I started eating a more consistent high fiber and high protein diet that I started to lift regularly. I met with a trainer at my local Planet Fitness and he directed me to lift 2-3 times per week with one session for each of the primary muscle groups. My weekly plan was:

1. Monday: Chest and Back

2. Wednesday: Shoulders and Arms

3. Friday: Legs and Core

Back to my story, the trainer had me doing workouts that would cover my entire body throughout the week and it would make me feel as if I wouldn't be able to walk during the weekends. However, despite my body feeling like it was broken, I was enjoying the experience. I knew that I was finally going to start losing weight and be on the road to a healthier me.

It wasn't easy, but I successfully lost weight through lifting weights.

To keep it really simple, check out this post on Nerd Fitness for how to build your own workout routine: http://bit.ly/1WPqCj6. I love this article because it helps you to find a place to start, and it targets your entire body. Definitely check it out if you're thinking about getting serious about starting a lifting routine. I will share some workouts later on in this chapter, but if you're wanting to get started on an all inclusive strength training routine, you can do no better than to follow the advice given at Nerd Fitness.

Whenever you think something isn't doable or will be too hard, just remember that you don't have to lift all the weights in the world. No one is expecting you to be able to show up at the gym and set a world record. The people at the gym that have a lot of muscle are that way for a reason. They have been crushing it for years. They didn't wake up one day with the Hulk's pecs. They have dedicated themselves to going to the gym and honing their craft.

Who knows, one day you might find yourself looking into the mirror and being met with the smile of someone who quite frankly looks amazing.

How Weight Lifting Helps Weight Loss

Lifting aids in weight loss for several reasons, but it's important to remember that at the end of the day muscle weighs more than fat. The scale will only tell you so much. Your level of fitness does not depend on that number on the scale. A better measurement is your waist in inches, or even just how you feel when looking into the mirror.

That being said, lifting weights aids in burning off a lot of excess fat. This is for several reasons:

- You burn calories during your recovery period in addition to the calories burned doing the actual workout. Your metabolism is on red alert and is more active because your body is working harder to repair muscles. This means that your efforts in the gym are paying dividends while you're eating dinner, while you're brushing your teeth, and even while you're sleeping. Cardio only burns calories while it's being performed.

- Regular weight lifting can have a dramatically positive effect on your mood, which keeps you coming back for more.

- It's easier to see results sooner. When you look at your body in the mirror and start to see muscles bulging, it really helps you to keep going!

- Weight lifting requires focus, which keeps your mind on what it's doing. This can aid in reducing stress levels, which is a plus in anyone's book. Some research suggests that being more mindful of our activities can aid in the effectiveness of the program.

The Best Strength Training Exercises to Lose Weight

The best strength training exercises are the ones that work for you. If you have a bad ankle like I do, you're not going to be doing one-legged squats using your bad leg. You need to find a workout that is going to push you, but also not leave you lying on the floor in agony either.

Listed below are 5 important strength-training workouts that you can try. Most of them seem difficult at first, but once you figure them out they really aren't too bad. For the easiest way to learn each workout, I have included a link to a Youtube video for each of the exercises so you can see them in action.

1. Squats
   - http://bit.ly/1UqPrV1
2. Deadlift
   - http://bit.ly/1WPqDne
3. Bench Press
   - http://bit.ly/1UqPv7f
4. Shoulder Press
   - http://bit.ly/1REwIEJ
5. Barbell Row
   - http://bit.ly/1MqL9tL

These are just a few workouts to get you started. Good luck in your strength training journey and remember to take it slow, take your time, and be consistent!

With bulging muscles and surges of energy pulsing through him the Fiber Guardian hurled his dumbbell up into the sky. The gauntlet was being thrown down as another enemy stepped forth. This hulking terror, this unearthly deluge of discouragement, filled the air with a blood curdling cry of "Submit Fiber Guardian, SUBMIT! You cannot lose weight! You cannot reach your goals!!" At first, fear creeped into FG's mind, but shortly thereafter he burst forward, grabbing the 20 foot behemoth by its thick neck and hoisting it over his shoulders. "To the abyss with you foul beast!" And with that, the Fiber Guardian destroyed Depresso once and for all with a great toss into the oblivion.

Tactic #19 Interval Training

Interval training is the bread and butter of workouts in the present day. It's a way to get more bang for your buck and save time in a busy day. Many studies have shown that interval training is actually much more effective for weight loss than traditional exercise. There is a lot of science that goes behind this, and frankly some of it is a little bit beyond my own comprehension.

The bottom line is that doing high intensity interval training, also known as HIIT, is one of the best ways you can speed up your weight loss progress.

My Story with Intervals

I can't honestly say where I first learned about intervals. It could have been from a friend or I could have read about it online. Regardless of where I learned it from, I went to gym one day about a year after college and decided to try it out. Turns out, I loved running in periods of intervals much better than just straight out running or biking.

Throughout college and the years after I still spent a fair amount of time just doing the bicycle at the gym. I enjoyed spinning and reading while I did my workout. I usually did about half an hour or 45 minutes and then called it a day. It took me awhile to realize that while it was great that I was getting out and going to the gym, what I was focusing on at the gym had to change. I couldn't keep going there, getting on the bike for a bit, stretching, and then going home and expecting mind-blowing results. It just wasn't going to happen unless I upped my game.

That is when intervals came along. I chose to run intervals on the treadmill (you can do intervals on other machines too), with 2 minutes of rest and 1 minute of hard effort. It gave me ample time to recover, and the minute was just long enough that I would feel really winded.

I aimed for about 30 minutes of this intense training, and the time always flew by. I was so focused on the time counting down for each section of my workout that I didn't have time to think, "Oh man when is this going to be over with!?" I was enjoying my time on the treadmill and enjoying the fact that I was trying something new.

I never would have believed it if someone told me that interval training would be one of the easier ways to workout (easy is a relative term here). However, I found that pushing myself for a small period of time and then allowing myself rest was a perfect way to workout. Anyone can do anything for a minute, and a minute of all out intense running is all it takes (provided you do that minute over and over again!).

I still enjoy running intervals to this day and find that it's one of the most beneficial and exciting ways to workout. I do HIIT on the treadmill, on a stair stepper machine, or even outside. Regardless of the "how," just remember that pushing yourself and reaching your highest potential is the real goal. It doesn't matter if the person next to you is blazing trails like they are running from a wildebeest. Everyone starts somewhere and works their way up.

How Intervals Are Beneficial for Weight Loss

Intervals can assist with weight loss in many ways. It worked for me personally and it can work for you too. Here are a few of those ways:

1. The body's metabolic rate increases after the workout for up to 24 hours. This is similar to weightlifting in that the body is unable to anticipate what is coming next, making it take longer to recover. Longer recovery times means that your body is burning more calories over time in order to bring your systems back on track. This is a good thing for those that are trying to lose weight.

2. Fat oxidation in the muscles increases and this aids in weight loss.

3. Intervals can be a lot more fun to do over the long run than traditional exercise. It's hard to get bored when you're constantly changing the parameters on your workout.

4. It can be a good pair to strength training as too much cardio can actually hinder muscle growth.

5. Because it takes less time to complete HIIT, training is great for those with busy lifestyles who want to get out of the gym quickly or reduce their workout time.

6. HIIT is great for your heart because it pushes you to the max, but doesn't keep you there long enough to do any damage.

How to do Intervals

Here are a few steps to make the most out of your interval training sessions:

- Choose your preferred machine or method of doing interval training. You can do intervals with just about any kind of cardio machine, including the treadmill, stationary bike, or stair stepper. Or you can skip the machines and do interval training at home through plyometric workouts or by going for a run outside.

- Start out slow. There is no sense in going to the gym, cranking the treadmill up to its max speed and falling off and breaking your face. DON'T DO THAT. Instead, warm up for at least 5 minutes, and then work your way up. Start with a medium speed, do that for a minute, and see how your body reacts.

- Once you feel comfortable, perform these workouts at the highest speed you can possibly do for one minute at a time. You want to be breathing really hard and really feeling it. If you end the minute and you can still talk to someone in a full sentence without taking a breath it's time to up your game and push yourself harder.

- Do the all out pace for 1 minute and then rest for two. Don't stop completely and lie on the floor for those 2 minutes, but don't push yourself hard at all during these two minutes. Let your body recover and get ready to do it all over again. If you can shorten the time to one minute on and one minute off, more power to you.

- To get the full benefit of HIIT training you need to push yourself to at least 90% of your top speed for that one minute.

- There is really no need to go any longer than 30 minutes when you're first starting out. You will feel the difference. The first few weeks after I started doing interval training I felt knocked out the next day. It really takes a lot out of you. Not to worry though, as this doesn't last long. If you're always exhausted the day after intervals, pull back and build up more slowly.

Start incorporating intervals into your workouts using these tips and you'll definitely start to see some results. Better yet, you'll start to have even more fun with weight loss and exercising in general. The more you try new things and the more you push yourself, the more you'll find yourself on the road to victory in your weight loss battle.

Tactic #20 Bodyweight Exercises

I love bodyweight exercises. I'm more excited about writing this chapter than most of the chapters in this book. Bodyweight exercises are useful, easy, and effective. First, let me explain how it worked for me.

My Story with Bodyweight Exercises

When I used to work out of the office for most of the day, I made it a habit to try to move around as often as possible. I even built myself a standing desk so that I wouldn't have to sit around all day (more on the standing desk in tactic #21). I knew that the sedentary lifestyle would kill me. No number of stretches, workouts, or massages from my lovely wife could ease the pain that resided in my lower back. Nothing could counteract the strain of sitting at work all day doing nothing.

Once I realized the problem I knew that I had to do something about it. I really enjoyed my job and quitting wasn't an option. I had to find a way to stay active while at work.

This is where bodyweight exercises came into play. During my breaks I would do push ups, calf raises, and squats in order to raise my heart rate and stretch my muscles. It was an excellent way to get my blood flowing in a short amount of time. At the end of the day I would feel much less stiff. Mentally, I felt better because my body was a little sore; not in the "I sat all day and didn't do a thing kind of way," but in the "Ouch those pushups were tough" kind of way.

Bodyweight exercises are one of the easiest ways to workout.

1. You can do them just about anywhere.

2. They take as much or as little time as you want them to.

3. You don't need any special equipment, because you are the equipment.

To this day I try to do as many small workouts throughout the day as I can in order to keep my body stretched and continually burning calories. This may be hard for some of you who don't have a private office space, but the idea is to get creative, and to not worry about what other people think. Easier said than done, but remember that other saying: if there's a will, there's a way!

> BONUS: Check out this PDF I created for ten tips for staying active at work: http://bit.ly/1Tae2vV. Print it out and put it near your computer for a good reminder!

The Many Benefits of Doing Bodyweight Exercises

Exercising with bodyweight exercises is awesome for several reasons. Here are just a few of them:

- It costs nothing to perform a bodyweight exercise. Even if you don't even own a single pair of workout clothing or equipment, bodyweight exercises can be completed free of charge.

- You can burn fat fast. With even just a few minutes of bodyweight training your metabolism is boosted. This is due to the afterburn effect, which helps you continue to burn calories after the workout has been completed.

- It's difficult to injure yourself doing bodyweight exercises because you can get used to the movements without putting any added strain on your body. You are used to being able to move around your own weight, so the chances of injuring yourself is very low.

- It's super fun to do at work. It gets you pumped up and ready to go back into the action, whatever that action might be.

- Bodyweight exercises can be challenging for anyone, regardless of fitness level. You can modify them to fit what you can do. Maybe you need to do pushups on your knees? Or maybe you can easily do a one legged squat? No problem! You only have to do what you're comfortable with.

- Most bodyweight exercises engage the core in some form, and this is very important to your overall level of fitness. The core is where we get our balance; a strong core reduces your chances of getting an injury.

- Bodyweight exercises are a great stress reliever that can be done just about anywhere.

- Weight loss is achieved through continual use of different bodyweight exercises. You don't have to go to the gym every day to have a great body; you can do workouts at home to reach a higher level of fitness.

- Bodyweight exercises are one of the easiest ways to start working out, while being able to achieve great results.

25 Bodyweight Exercises to Try

Now that you know what bodyweight exercises can do for you, here are some of the best ones to try. Choose a few of these, try them, master them, and then try some more. Before you know it, you'll be able to complete ten of these workouts in about 10-15 minutes for a really good boost in your day.

In each of these workouts, you'll find a link to a video that demonstrates how to do them. I have found that just reading about how to do an exercise isn't very helpful, so I think it much more prudent to link out videos for you.

1. Regular Pushups: http://bit.ly/1XTM46S

2. Desk Pushups: http://bit.ly/1MHSvDS

3. Diamond Pushups: http://bit.ly/1MHSsZ0

4. Jumping Jacks: http://bit.ly/1RrgGsl

5. Sit-Ups: http://bit.ly/1RrgEkd

6. Crunches: http://bit.ly/1q6Qpsv

7. Bicycle Crunch: http://bit.ly/1pClyDD

8. Squats: http://bit.ly/1UqPrV1

9. Lunges: http://bit.ly/1LO6kGa

10. Burpees: http://bit.ly/21LmUIs

11. Planks: http://bit.ly/21LmT7g

12. Side Plank: http://bit.ly/1ocpUQY

13. Wall sit: http://bit.ly/1q6Qvk1

14. Single leg deadlift: http://bit.ly/1MHSGzc

15. Step-up: http://bit.ly/1WPr9BB

16. Calf raise: http://bit.ly/1XTMj1y

17. Crab-walk: http://bit.ly/1RsVxAk

18. Superman: http://bit.ly/1UqPWi1

19. Chair-dips: http://bit.ly/1RrgWaI

20. Arm-circles: http://bit.ly/1MqLxZc

21. Hip-raises: http://bit.ly/1pClJyI

22. Dumbbell rows (you can use anything, even a milk jug!): http://bit.ly/1MqLz3b

23. Bear Crawl: http://bit.ly/1Scetks

24. Mountain Climber: http://bit.ly/1UPC1Bw

25. Back Bridge: http://bit.ly/1RVbn4G

Practical Tips for Doing Bodyweight Exercises

1. Like anything, do bodyweight exercises in moderation. Three hundred pushups in one day would be awesome, but that might become boring and potentially dangerous for you if you do it every day.

2. Vary your exercises. Try to get good workouts for your legs, chest, back, arms, and core. Be sure to spend just as much time in one muscle group as you do in others to prevent injury. Don't forget leg day!

3. Take it slow when you're just starting out, especially when you're not sure how to do an exercise.

4. If you can, ask a friend to watch your form (or use a mirror) and be sure to correct it as bad form can do more harm than good.

5. Above all, always remember to listen to your body and to stop if you start to feel too much pain. That twentieth squat isn't worth it if you have to spend weeks recovering from a pulled hamstring.

Tactic #21: Use a Standing Desk

Sitting all day can kill you. It even has its own disease name, aptly called "sitting disease." Living a sedentary lifestyle—sitting in a desk all day at work only to come back and veg out in front of the TV—is one of the reasons why many Americans find themselves obese. On its own, watching too much TV has been linked to an increased chance of contracting heart disease, and we can only guess that this is largely due to the fact that most of us aren't watching TV from the comfort of a treadmill.

Utilizing a standing desk is a major life change that will give you positive results. The benefits I obtained from standing for most of my work day were huge, and it's one of the best decisions that I could have made when trying to lose weight. I find that the simple act of standing changed my life in positive ways, and it's one that I cannot wait to share with you. Let's start by building the desk!

How to Build A Standing Desk

I recommend building a standing desk because it's actually super easy. If you're not mechanically inclined, get a friend to build one for you. If you have more money than time, buy one, but keep in mind that standing desks are very expensive. There are some really interesting and effective mechanical standing desks that can be adjusted with a push of a button.

If you're like me, you'll opt to make your own. Here's how I did it for just about 30 bucks using Ikea parts. I followed the instructions from this site (http://bit.ly/1Sm9dwY). Their instructions are super clear and very helpful. The only thing I did different is to buy the Ikea parts online because I did not have a store near me.

It will look like this when you're done (with or without the messy desk!).

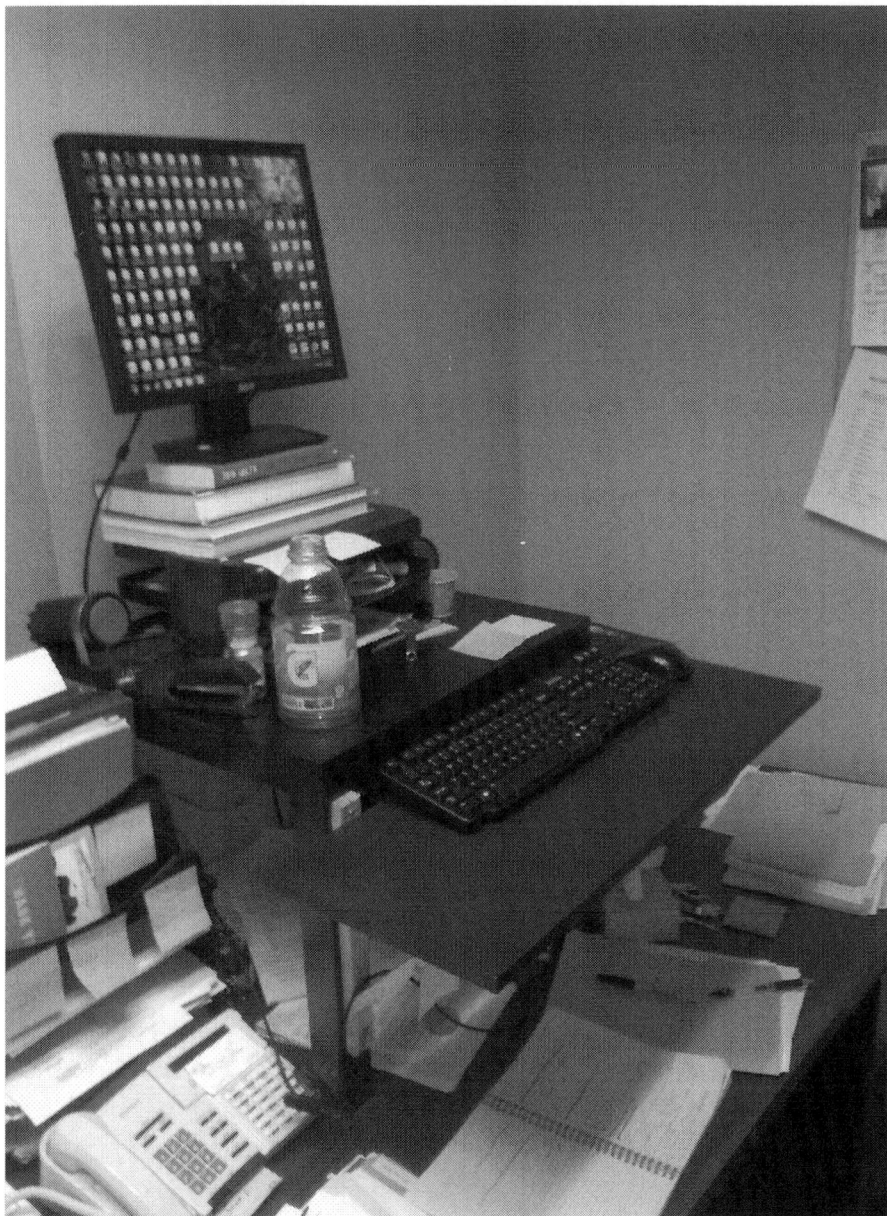

The Benefits of Standing

Standing was a great change for me, and not just because of the confidence boost I received every time someone complimented my cool-looking standing desk. Here are a few of the ways using a standing desk benefited me:

- Standing more during the day decreased my lower back pain. After spending a year sitting most of the day my lower back was letting me have it! Going to the gym, doing yoga, and stretching every which way would not completely relieve the pain. Amazingly, within one week of utilizing a standing desk my lower back pain was gone. I haven't had back pain that intense ever since.

- I was able to burn a lot more calories from standing most of the day as opposed to sitting. To see how many more calories you can burn check out this handy dandy calculator: http://bit.ly/1pNHP22.

- The way that I arranged my office meant that I could alternate between standing and sitting. Even too much of a good thing can end up being a bad thing and standing all day isn't good either. I spent a good part of the day on the computer utilizing my standing desk and I was able to sit down and do paperwork, take phone calls, and talk to people that came into my office. It ended up being a really good mix of sitting and standing.

- I felt much better physically and mentally at the end of the day, My back pain was gone and my brain felt much more active. I didn't feel like I needed to take an afternoon nap every day!

- I personally think that standing was a major boon in continuing my weight loss journey because it promoted activity throughout the day.

Practical Tips for Standing More Than you Sit

It's important to remember several things when utilizing a standing desk:

1. Mix up standing and sitting as it promotes even more movement.

2. Make sure that the height of the desk is appropriate for you. A desk too high or too low could cause other problems for your back and your arms!

3. Don't be fooled into thinking that standing all day gives you the right to skip out on other physical activities. No sir! it's a great tactic to combat the sedentary lifestyle but is not a means of exercise.

4. You can stand at home too! Build yourself a standing desk to use at home instead of sitting in front of the computer or the tv!

5. Stand as much as you can and sit only when you need to.

In the end, utilizing a standing desk is an excellent way to combat sitting disease. Make this tactic a priority if you have an office job, and don't worry about what other people think. You are making a positive life choice and should not feel ashamed, even if it brings unwanted attention to you. Stand and be proud to stand!

The enemy's smirk disappeared in an instant. Lackadaisical, the defender of lethargy and the champion of laziness had taken notice of new developments within his domain. As he looked down at the office space, what he thought was his crowning accomplishment in his efforts to keep people obese, he was stricken with terror. This creature, this Fiber Guardian, or whatever he called himself was standing. STANDING at work! Oh the outrage! Oh the horror! Lackadaisical growled at the cosmos and swore to himself that no matter how many tactics the Fiber Guardian mastered, he would never win the war. In his cockiness the enemy calmed, knowing that time was his ally, and that opportunities would present themselves in the most delicious of ways.

Section 4

LOW-STRESS LIVING

Let me tell you the story of a caveman named Nadroj:

The year is 40000 BC. Nadroj the caveman is just waking up from his restless sleep of the night before. The structure he dwells in is relatively safe, but he still sleeps in fear of a greater predator finishing him off. As he grabs his makeshift spear and wanders off in search of small game, he wonders if this will be the last day he gets to see the sunrise.

The day's hunt is unsuccessful. As the miles fade away under his tiring feet, Nadroj starts to turn for home with no food and no water nearby. He realizes a moment later that he has gone too far for one day. He is nowhere near home and the sun is setting. Such a mistake could prove disastrous.

He starts to run for home. He knows that no man is capable of surviving on his own without shelter in the wild and dangerous world. The lands Nadroj has ventured into are filled with creatures much bigger than him. He has to move fast if he wanted to make it out of the predator's territory before dark.

His heart beats rapidly as terrifying memories of his brother Nimrod being ripped apart race through his mind. He runs as fast as a man can run.

It is dark when he finally finds his way home. Luckily he is safe and unharmed today, although very hungry. He drinks some of his remaining water supply and a few berries and lies down to sleep. Dreams of the next day assault him and his sleep is restless.

The next day will be even harder as he is running very low on food. Alas, this is the life of poor Nadroj, and survival is all that matters to him.

Stress has been around since the dawn of man and it has taken on many different forms. One thing for certain is that stress nowadays affects us in very similar ways (elevated heart rate, nervousness), while the cause of that stress has continually changed. Stress used to be invoked by predatory beasts and now it's now caused by crappy jobs and credit card bills.

We obviously don't live in fear of being eaten like in the above story, but we live with stress nonetheless. We worry day to day about paying the bills, our children's education, our parents' health, and a hundred other troubles.

So what's the difference between stressed Nadroj and stressed you?

Well, the difference is huge and not subtle. Nadroj combated his stress with running and jumping and moving this way and that. He had to! Nowadays, humans combat stress with fatty foods and television. The vast majority of us don't run to the gym in order to de-stress. We run to the fridge and grab the first delicious thing we see.

Where Nadroj runs, we snack. This isn't because we are awful human beings. Not at all! It's because this path is the path of least resistance to get an immediate fix and to feel better and reduce stress. If Nadroj didn't have to hunt to eat, he'd probably be just as lazy as we are.

We in the first world face a very different challenge than anybody from prehistoric times. We can choose to be lazy and still survive for long periods of time. We don't need to be fit in order to run away from predators or to catch ourselves dinner. Yes, achieving a level of fitness does keep us away from the doctor and in generally better health, but fitness is not something we absolutely NEED to survive. Yes, being fit does give us a better chance at a long and happy life, but it isn't necessary for immediate survival in most cases.

Due to this, we have to *choose* to reduce our stress levels and lose weight. It's something we have to push for and fight for constantly. We don't have the luxury of running away from huge predators, and we don't have to lift rocks and trees in order to build a shelter. We have to make living a healthier life a priority that we strive for each and every day.

Making Stress Reduction a Goal

Everyone struggles with stress. The story above demonstrates that stress is not something we can avoid completely no matter where we find ourselves in life. We all find ourselves in tough spots in our lives.

Choosing to do nothing will certainly not help your stress levels and your symptoms of stress will only get worse. Unfortunately, in this day and age, you have to make some difficult choices and fight hard to reduce your stress levels. You cannot totally rely on natural forces and a "normal" way of life if you want to stay happy and stress free.

Personally, I battled stress throughout my journey, and I still battle it. I'm an anxious person by nature and I struggle with stress daily. However, by utilizing all of the tactics in this book, my stress is much lower and it's manageable now. Between going to the gym, drinking green tea, and focusing on getting enough sleep at night, I'm in a much better spot.

I can tell you honestly that reducing my stress levels has played a major part in my weightloss journey, and I hope you find this section extremely helpful, informative, and practical.

Stress Reduction Tactics

Keep in mind that there are many different ways to reduce stress, but the tactics that made it into this book are the ones that worked for me and that I have found particularly effective.

1. Practice yoga
2. Reduce boredom
3. Find a project
4. Sleep more
5. Focus on breathing through meditation
6. Get a pet
7. Get rid of a bad habit
8. Drink tea
9. Listen to music

Reducing Stress For Weight Loss

Stress cause changes to our body that, if not dealt with, can cause us many problems down the line. Stress affects weight gain in many ways:

- Binge eating and emotional eating

- Weakened immune system which causes all sorts of problems as it's much easier to avoid the gym or overeat if you have a cold.

- When over-stressed the body creates higher levels of the hormone called cortisol, which increases our appetite.

- Being stressed can interrupt our sleep patterns by reducing the amount of sleep we get, thus creating a bad cycle of exhaustion and stressful days.

- It's harder to calm the mind when stressed and it's harder to focus on important tasks, which only adds to our stress levels!

Stress is an important factor in your weight-loss journey. It's one that you need to deal with and quickly. If you don't have a plan for reducing stress in your life, chances are you might already be too stressed! But don't worry, it isn't too late. Follow the tactics I'm going to lay out here, and you'll be well on your way to achieving victory in the face of stress and ultimately succeeding in your weight loss journey.

Tactic #22: Practice Yoga for Stress Reduction

Of all the ways to reduce stress, doing yoga is one of the best. Yoga allows time and space for your mind to reach a state of peace while your body is being stretched to the max. I know this because I have experienced that peace that comes at the end of doing a yoga session, when you just finish the final pose and get to just lie there on the mat. This feeling of peace is unsurpassed by any other activity, and it truly feels good for the mind, body, and soul.

Yoga is one of the most innovative, calming, and uplifting ways to spend your evening. Practicing it means reaching towards mindfulness and having a deeper understanding of what is going on in your head.

Yoga focuses on the breath. Every movement is paired with the breath. This pairing helps you to achieve a state of calm through breathing and then focusing on the breath. I recommend yoga to anyone that leads a high-stress lifestyle and needs a good outlet for that stress.

Yoga is not just simply of means of relaxing, though. Quite the contrary, yoga is a serious workout, and even Tony Horton from P90X has dedicated an entire day's workout to the practice. Lest you think yoga is akin to an easy Sunday morning walk, think again.

My Story with Yoga

In one of the yoga videos I use on Amazon Prime, the instructor constantly brings it back to "focusing on the breath." Many of of the stretches come "from the heart" which encourages you to open up your body as well as your mind.

While I do not practice it weekly (and actually yoga is most productive when it's completed several times per week), even doing yoga once in awhile feels great. I can attest that my system calms down and I feel at peace right away. All of the worries and troubles that I have melt away during the routine.

I also found that yoga was extremely easy to do. All you really need is a comfy floor or a yoga mat (which I happened to already own; if you don't they are only 5 bucks at 5 Below). Lay out your mat and search for a yoga video on Youtube, Amazon Video, Netflix, or another streaming service. If you like to rock it old school, pop in a VHS tape. You could even join a yoga class and get the proper instruction. Yoga is extremely popular nowadays, and more than likely there is a yoga class that is meeting somewhere very close to you. Just type in "yoga near me" into google and you'll probably find a suitable studio within driving distance.

I've never taken a yoga class myself, but I have done many different yoga videos, including the P90X yoga (if you want an INTENSE yoga session I recommend that one). I enjoy doing yoga in the comfort of my own home, but I wouldn't mind doing it in a class as well. Either way you want to do it, it truly is a good practice to get into.

The Many Benefits of Yoga

Practicing yoga brings with it a slew of benefits, not the least of which is that it can help you to reduce stress. Here are some of the many benefits that you can expect to achieve, whether you become a regular yoga participant or a casual one.

- The most obvious benefit of practicing yoga is that it increases your flexibility. This is important to reduce potential sports-related injuries. Flexibility also helps to reduce back pain.

- Yoga is a full body workout that strengthens multiple muscles at once. This is great to achieve an overall high level of fitness as it increases balance and control.

- Yoga reduces stress by limiting levels of the stress hormone cortisol.

- Blood flow increases when doing yoga which aids in increasing circulation to your hands and your feet.

- Yoga improves sleep because it helps the nervous system to calm down, relaxing mind and body while giving you a solid workout. Sounds like a win-win to me!

- Yoga increases the effectiveness of your immune system.

- IBS and other digestive-related issues are helped by yoga, mainly because yoga helps to reduce stress. Some people that practice yoga also suspect that some of the twisting poses may aid in moving waste through the system faster, although this has not yet been tested.

- Practicing yoga eases pain. Whether you deal with back pain, joint pain, or carpal tunnel, yoga is a great way to reduce the pain.

There are many more benefits to practicing yoga, but these are some of the most relevant. Try it out for yourself and you'll notice the difference.

Tips for Practicing Yoga

1. Yoga can be practiced individually or with a friend. However, if you do practice with a friend, be sure to keep the talking to a minimum. Yoga is meant to be a spiritual and introspective time. Constant interruptions disturb the flow.

2. Find a good place to do yoga that is comfortable and free of distractions. This can be outside on your deck, inside where it's warm, or on top of the roof. Anywhere that puts your mind at ease is a great place to practice.

3. When practicing, fall within yourself and follow the instructor on the journey. Don't worry about life or all of the other things that are stressing you out. Focus on the breath and focus on what your body is doing. As Master Yoda says, "Control, you must learn control!" (If you were doing yoga, wouldn't you want Master Yoda as your instructor!? I know I would.)

4. Just like I have had fun writing this book, be sure you're having fun when doing yoga. If you hate it, consider moving on to another activity that you actually do like! But do me a favor and give it a chance; I have a feeling you'll love it.

5. Most importantly, just remember that you won't be able to do all of the poses when you're starting out. Take your time and learn as much as you can!

Tactic #23: Kick Boredom to the Curb and Find a Hobby

According to Merriam Webster, boredom is "the state of being weary and restless through lack of interest." I would expand that to include that feeling bored means that your current state of mind is less than ideal and that you're not happy.

This tactic is about reducing the amount of times you find yourself bored, thereby helping you to avoid eating cookies because you don't know what else to do with yourself.

Similar to tactic #15 (find something active that you love to do), tactic #23 is all about finding hobbies that you love to do. The difference with this tactic is that the hobby doesn't have to be a physically active hobby. Yep, that's right! It can be anything that helps you to stay busy, fight boredom, and ultimately reduce stress.

Wait, I'll take that back for a second. It can be anything that isn't scarfing down donuts or going on a Netflix binge. The hobby needs to meet a few criteria in order to count under this tactic:

1. The hobby needs to be something you love to do. You need to be able to look forward to it, or you might not want to do it.

2. The hobby shouldn't be detrimental to your weight loss journey. This means the hobby shouldn't be competitive pie eating or sumo wrestling.

3. The hobby shouldn't cause any extra stress. That's what we're trying to avoid here!

The importance of this tactic is to take your mind off whatever it is that ails you and to help you focus on more important things. The hobby should be such that the stress of life cannot enter. Your mind is so enraptured by what you're doing that it loses its connection to anxiety.

The Fiber Guardian's Favorite Hobbies

I love to stay busy. Even on my days off I can only watch TV for so long. My limit's pretty much one good movie every once in awhile, and even then I have a hard time sitting still through it. (Unless it's Lord of The Rings, Star Wars, or Star Trek. I would watch those movies any day!)

I have found that staying busy and finding enjoyment in hobbies has been huge for my weight loss journey. It's super easy to feel stressed when you're bored. The weight of the world can easily crush down on your shoulders if that's all you have to think about.

Even the busiest people get bored once in awhile. Finding productive ways to spend down time is paramount to avoiding the negative side effects of boredom.

Some of the hobbies I enjoy include:

- Working on my Fiber Guardian blog – Seriously, this has been one of the best hobbies I could have ever gotten into because it's a long-term project.

- Writing this book.

- Reading – I say reading, but I do most of my "reading" by listening to Amazon Audible books.

- Playing sports of all different kinds.

- Going on walks with my wife. We love to walk, and recently we have been finding some excellent greenways in North Carolina.

- Board games – Board games are super fun to play with your significant other or with a big group. With this hobby you get the added benefit of hanging with friends and enjoying good company. Whether you're playing party games like Catchphrase or more serious strategy board games like Lords of Waterdeep, getting into board games is a great hobby.

- Video games – Woah video games!? But you said not to be in front of the TV too long? True enough, but playing video games online with my brother who lives 18 hours away from me is a worthwhile hobby in my opinion. Try to avoid addicting games like World of Warcraft and you will be good to go. Anything in moderation of course.

These are just some of the hobbies I have gotten into over the past few years. I have found that looking forward to these activities instead of looking forward to food has made a huge difference for me. Sure, sometimes playing board games is fused with having a pizza party or a few beers, but the idea is that I was staying busy. I wasn't spending inordinate amounts of time watching netflix and eating chicken wings alone in the basement.

The Benefits of Decreasing Boredom

Boredom is not something we just want to actively avoid. It's something that can be dangerous to our health if we do not make it a goal to find something satisfying to do. Often, it's not even something we can control the moment it happens. We need to be wary of falling into boredom. Yes, we all need to take time to take a deep breath and relax, but we should also be careful not to spend hours upon hours vegging out on the couch.

According to the paper The Unengaged Mind, author John Eastwood posits that boredom can have several serious consequences. To name a few:

- Overeating

- Drug and alcohol abuse

- Depression and Anxiety

- Increased risk of making mistakes due to lack of focus and desire.

Boredom happens when our mind has a desire we cannot place. Thoughts like, "I just don't know what I want to do right now" enter the mind. Having a hobby counteracts these thoughts, and helps guides our time. It's hard to be bored when your friends are coming over for game night!

Decreasing boredom helps you to:

- Have something to look forward to

- Decrease levels of stress

- Have less down time that can turn into worrying

- Be a person of action by actively fighting for a productive life

- Become more focused (tactic #1). The less time you spend bored, the more time you'll have for more important activities. Everyone has experienced the dulling of the mind that occurs when feeling bored, and it's something we should actively avoid.

I will mention that on the flip side there are several people who say that boredom can actually be good for you. My stance is that continual boredom is good for no one. YES we need to be sure we are taking time to rest, reflect, and calm our minds, but we need not look to boredom to do that.

There are many people in this world that are just way too busy and don't need a hobby. There are also those who don't have enough to do and find themselves home alone too often. This tactic is merely meant as a way to share that being involved in hobbies is beneficial, and much better than alternative of constant boredom.

Practical Steps to Find the Perfect Hobby

There are so many different hobbies out there that you could start right now if you wanted to. I could list them out for you, but there are way too many to list. Here is a good site called Discover A Hobby (http://bit.ly/1RBJ36c) and it can help you to find a hobby that you love.

Keep in mind the following tips:

1. Don't be afraid to try something new. Who knows? You might find one that you love!

2. If you find that your activity is causing boredom, drop it and find something else. Even if the hobby is serving other people, if you don't find that it brings you enjoyment it's not something that you will be able to do long-term, and you won't be able to give 100% to it.

3. The more people involved the better. Being involved with other people in a community is really good for us and being around others makes it very hard to be bored!

4. If you find that your activity isn't helping you reach your weight loss goals, or is even causing you to backtrack, find a new hobby!

Regardless of how you choose to spend your time, remember to take the time to rest as well. Just not so much time that boredom finds a hold!

Laughing joyously the Fiber Guardian wrote about saving the world from being fiber deficient. Boredom would find no hold on him and his arch nemesis Lackadaisical had lost yet another battle. In the attempt to defeat the Fiber Guardian with restlessness, he had inadvertently divulged another tactic that would ultimately spell his demise...

Tactic #24: Get Involved: Find a Project

Finding a project is more than just a tactic to keep yourself busy. It's a way to keep yourself motivated, happy, and stress-free. The sense of completion at the end of a good project is merely the icing on the cake. The journey to get to the finish line is truly the core of why having a project is so good for you, especially when that journey was difficult.

It may seem counterintuitive to add more "work" to your plate if you have a busy job, a family, and other commitments. However, having a project that is above and beyond the normal day-to-day is huge for reducing stress. It gives you something to look forward to, something that will make you feel really good about spending time on it.

Who among us has ever finished a Netflix binge and said, "I'm SO glad I just did that. I feel great and I feel so accomplished!"

Doesn't sound familiar? No?

Then do something that matters and get involved!

My idea of a project is anything that you do that takes a lot of work and demands constant attention over time. You do not necessarily have to lead the project, but you need to be invested in the end goal. The project doesn't have to take years, and it doesn't have to be world changing, but it does need to occupy your time and then leave you with a satisfying sense of accomplishment.

The Fiber Guardian's Projects

The following are some great projects that you could do to reduce stress and find fulfilment. I have found these projects to be both fun and give an uplifting sense of accomplishment at their completion:

- Work on a gift for a friend or family member. Create something from scratch out of wood, sew something, or make a necklace. Any of these DIY gift options will work: http://bit.ly/1URNpM7. For Christmas two years ago I created a present for my Dad by using a woodburner and a little bit of time. I put several quotes on it from one of my favorite movies of all time (Dead Poet's Society) and I even made a little stand for it out of popsicle sticks. It didn't cost an arm and a leg but the finished product was something we will both remember for a long time to come!

- Create your very own board game. This can be a very involved project but one that would be excellent for this tactic. It would take a while, but seeing the final product (and playing with it) would be amazing. Check out this article for a complete guide on how to make your own board game: http://bit.ly/1Pw8aWJ.

- Write a book. Writing this book has been an amazing project for me to have, and it has been one of the most in-depth and time-consuming things I have ever done. I know that when this book is out for the world to see it will become one of my greatest accomplishments, regardless of how well it does in sales.

- Make a blog. Besides writing this book, building my Fiber Guardian blog was one of the coolest projects I ever undertook. It's been around for about a year now and I enjoy every moment of time I get to spend working on it.

- Learn something new. Whether you're going for your master's or taking a course on Udemy, learning stretches our minds and causes us to grow. However, If you find yourself bored you might want to consider a new class!

How Working on a Project is Huge for Stress Reduction

Stress comes when you're feeling overwhelmed, unimportant, or overworked. Having a project that you're invested in and that you love counteracts all of these. Working on a project allows you to look forward to the completion of a job that you can be proud of. I was so excited to share my Dad's finished Christmas gift with him because I had put so much time into it. If I had just bought him a gift card I wouldn't have been nearly as excited to give him his present.

As discussed in the previous chapter, keeping busy and staying involved can reduce stress by not allowing you the time to dwell on negative parts of your life. Instead, your mind becomes intent on finishing the project and your mind is lit on fire (in a good way) with ideas on how to complete that project to the best of your ability.

Tips on Finding a Good Project

There are several ways to find a project:

1. Brainstorm by making a list of items and then mashing them up in order to find the perfect project for you:

   • Things you love to do.

   • Things you're good at.

   • Something that will help someone else out.

   • Something that you'll feel really good about on completion.

2. Join a local church in order to be involved with their community projects (blood drive, community Easter egg hunt, etc.). Beyond joining up with a community of people, you'll have many opportunities to improve your neighborhood! You can feel accomplished and satisfied that you're indeed making a difference.

3. If you're looking for a BIG project you could even join a local homeless shelter or soup kitchen and volunteer. You will have something you belong to and in this case it is something that really matters. Beyond your daily job, you're giving back to the community in a positive way. You may even discover your true passion!

Projects are an extremely effective way for anyone that is looking to reduce stress in their lives. Start one now and you'll begin to see the benefits for yourself.

Tactic #25: Sleep The Right Amount

Most of us can't afford to sleep as much as we'd like. If we could, many of us would choose to sleep between 9-10 hours every night. Unfortunately, the demands of life prevent us from living out our dreams of abundant sleep.

Sleeping too much can actually be a problem, but sleep deprivation is far more common than too much sleep.. It's common knowledge that just about 7-8 hours of sleep is what we should be aiming for every night, but of course, this is not always possible.

For example, how do new mothers and fathers get their sleep every night? The answer, plain and simple, is that they don't. They are forced to go without the required amount of sleep for many months, until their child's sleep patterns regulate. Parents survive this time, but it shows that it just isn't possible to get enough sleep every night.

Ask yourself the following questions and think about them throughout this chapter:

1. Do I get enough sleep every night?
2. What happens to me when I don't get enough sleep?
3. Do I even think about how much sleep I get or do I just brush it off and go about my life?
4. What steps am I taking to make sure I get enough sleep every night?

My Story with Sleep

Sleeping enough has been difficult at times throughout my life. I usually go to bed with enough time to get 6-8 hours of sleep. I know that if I get any less than 6 hours I will be exhausted, irritable, and won't function at my full potential. If I go several days with less than 6 hours, I can feel my body start to react negatively, and I know that if I keep that streak up it will only be a matter of time before I get sick.

During the initial period of my weight loss journey I knew I'd need to get on the right track with my sleep, especially since I would be lifting and working out at the gym. Those who workout are breaking the body down and expending a lot of energy and need more sleep to recover.

I made it a priority to get enough sleep at night, and this helped aid in my recovery, as well as giving me enough energy to go to work, and then the gym afterwards. Back then, I was working really late, which meant the gym would come later as well, making me even more tired. I'm a night owl, but a long day's work was taxing. However, I found that if I did get enough sleep the night before, everything went much more smoothly throughout the day!

Moreover, sleeping enough helped me to feel more calm. My stress levels decreased dramatically. It was amazing to me how much more positive I would be during the days that I slept 8 hours. The sun shone just a little bit brighter, and any problems I had seemed so much more beatable than they would have been if I were exhausted.

The Benefits of Getting Enough Sleep

Getting the right amount of sleep is paramount to a solid weight loss program. You can't have one without the other. While coffee is indeed a good weight loss tactic (#14) it cannot be used as a substitute for getting good sleep. Most Americans do not get enough sleep every night, and it's something that contributes greatly to the obesity epidemic.

Sleeping the right amount has plenty of health benefits that make it worth it to turn in early, and even hit the snooze button if you need to:

- You will be less likely to become irritable throughout the day.

- Sleeping repairs the body which helps to reduce the effects of a rough day.

- Stress is reduced because our body is able to heal overnight, and thus is more readily able to deal with the curve balls that life throws at us.

- We can solve problems better and our brains function at a higher level when we are rested. Our memory is boosted, our focus increases, and we are better able to make important decisions throughout the day.

- A good night's sleep can decrease anxiety levels, thereby reducing the toll that a "tough day at the office" costs us.

Of all of these good reasons to sleep, the goal of reducing stress is one of the most important because of how stress can spiral out of control. It can become a catch-22 if you're not careful. If you find yourself not getting enough sleep on a consistent basis your stress levels will rise and you'll have a hard time getting back on track and getting enough sleep because you're stressed! Don't find yourself in this cycle; be sure to get enough sleep!

How to Counteract Sleep Deprivation and Get Back On Track

Here are some practical tips to getting enough sleep each and every night.

1. Wear a sleep tracker like a Fitbit. There is no better way to see how you're doing with your sleep on a regular basis than having it examined via a sleep tracker (unless you join a sleep study).

2. Go to bed earlier. Obvious though it may be, going to bed early is something you have to start doing if you're serious about getting enough sleep every night.

3. Avoid eating meals too late. If you're hungry before you go to bed try drinking some water instead. Eating right before bed can keep you up, but it's also a really poor decision when trying to lose weight.

4. Before you climb into bed, turn the lights off and stretch for about 5-10 minutes. It will help you fall asleep faster.

5. Drinking herbal decaffeinated or caffeine-free tea right before you go to bed can calm your system and help you sleep better.

6. Sleep naked. Sleeping naked is actually much healthier for us as it helps to regulate our body temperature.

7. Get yourself a good set of blinds or a black shade to make the room completely dark. Darkness helps us to sleep better and longer without as many interruptions.

Know yourself and your body. Learn what your optimal sleep time is, as well as what sleep methods work for you. Basically, find what works and stick with it!

Sweet dreams Fiber Guardian. Sweet dreams of ultimate frisbee and walks on the beach...

Tactic #26: Breathe Deep and Meditate

How often per day do you stop to take a deep breath? One? Two? Twenty five?

If you're like most of the busy people out in the world, you might only stop to take a deep breath once in awhile or possibly not at all!

However, I suggest that you take more time to stop, breathe deep, and THEN continue along in your day. A deep breath can make all the difference in reducing your stress levels and keeping your mind focused on daily tasks.

One of the best ways to learn to focus on the breath is to learn more about meditation. Meditation is the practice of calming your mind in order to become more aware of your external surroundings and internal rumblings. It's a practice that forces you to take deep breaths, sit still, and think.

Meditation is for everyone, even those who can't sit still for long (like me!) and those who are very busy. The idea, like all of the tactics in this book, is to improve in one small way in order to reduce stress. Beating stress is not easy, and I want you to be as prepared as possible in order to better defend against the constant onslaught of stress.

My Story with Meditation and Deep Breathing

I don't spend hours every day in a robe, sitting cross-legged in my living room. I bet that is the image that comes to your mind when reading about meditation, but I can assure you that I'm not a monk. I have found meditation useful in that it forces me to be quiet, think, and to pray. I choose to pray to God as He is my higher power, but prayer is not required for meditation to work. Even just sitting still and thinking positive thoughts can do wonders for my mood.

I'm not an expert at meditation, but at a basic level, I have found that quieting my mind and avoiding external stimuli helps me to slow down.

Taking quiet time allows me to become more in touch with my feelings. Meditation allows me that time to think, "Wow, I really wasn't helpful to my wife today, but now I know what I could have done better."

I usually only do it for 15 or 20 minutes, but even that small amount of time can make a world of difference. Afterwards I'm better able to respond to situations appropriately and can see the next step to solving a problem more clearly.

It might be hard to locate the time and energy to sit still, but trust me, doing so will definitely reduce your stress levels, and will ultimately assist you in your weight loss journey.

How Meditation and Deep Breathing Help to Reduce Stress

Along the way I discovered several benefits to deep breathing and meditation:

- Meditation increases focus. Not only does this aid in tactic #1, it also helps to keep you moving towards your goals. The muck clears and the steps that you need to take to reach your goal crystalize.

- Meditation reduces relationship stress by helping you to respond better to co-workers, family members, and significant others. Practicing meditation forces you to respond more slowly. Ultimately your level of patience will rise. Let's face it, people do pretty stupid things almost every day! With a clear mind, you can more effectively handle these situations with grace and compassion for the other person, because you know that you have bad days as well.

- The self-awareness that is gained through self-reflection is an easy way to reduce stress. You're able to become more aware of WHY you're feeling a certain way, and thus you're able to figure out the next best steps to feel better. Sometimes the answer is as simple as needing more sleep, or recognizing that you're cranky and that is why your spouse's comment bothered you so much.

- Calming your mind means calming your body as the body and mind go hand in hand.

Practical Meditation Steps

Meditation is actually a fairly easy thing to do if you take it slow. If you put a half hour timer on, go into a dark room, and try to quiet your mind, it will feel like hours. Like every tactic in this book, the idea is to start slow and work your way up consistently!

The first step is taking the time to do it; the second step is being determined to get better at it. Meditation may not come easily to you. You might need to spend a few sessions to really understand how to make it work for you. Just remember to make time for it, and then determine if it's something that you want as part of your daily routine.

Here are some steps you can take to begin your meditation journey:

1. Start by meditating for just a few minutes per day. That's it! It's all about baby steps and making meditation a habit.

2. Be consistent! If you really want to get into meditation, create a chart for yourself and do at least a couple of minutes of deep breathing per day for a month. Once you start to do it regularly it will become a habit!

3. Pick one thought or phrase and focus on that during your meditation time. Try to resist all other thoughts and instead pour all of your mental energy into that phrase, thought, or idea of your choice.

4. Be aware of the wandering mind. Your thoughts will indeed wander and at first you'll be all over the place. "Why am I doing this!?" Why am I sitting here?" I'm wasting so much time…" Don't worry about this at all! If you're like me, this will be a common occurrence, and will happen repeatedly! Just bring your thoughts back to focus and stay there as long as you can.

5. Recognize that while clearing of the mind is the purpose of meditation, your mind will probably never be fully clear. It will always have some thoughts rolling around! Don't worry about it. Just try to come back and refocus on one idea.

6. Try asking yourself why you think the way that you do. This will lead to introspection and you'll start to learn more about yourself and the way that your mind works.

For a complete resource on this subject see Zen Habit's Meditation Guide: http://bit.ly/1Pw8jts.

Tactic #27: Find Fido (Get a Pet)

WHAT!? A dog will really reduce my stress levels? But that's so much work! It will be just another thing that I have to take care of!

First of all, cool your jets. I'm not saying you have to get a 100 pound dog that needs to go outside 4 times a day. You can get any kind of pet you want. You could even grow a cactus and call it your pet, although people might judge you. But really, even a simple plant would be a good way to start getting used to the idea of a pet.

The secret sauce of pet ownership is that it gives you something to take care of that is not yourself. Someone else (or something else if you get a plant) depends on you for its life to continue on. This is so huge that I have to say it again.

Someone else's well-being has been elevated above your own. You are unable to solely worry about yourself.

Pet owners see things in a fresh perspective which helps their own anxiety to go down.

I currently live and work in a retirement home, where we allow pets to stay with the residents. I personally get to see how much of a difference these animals can make in people's lives. It has been an eye opener for sure. I wouldn't have believed it as much as I do now, but pets can change people's lives for the better.

For example, we have one lady that loves her dog more than anything else. You can tell that Bear is one of her main reasons to keep on. She can't remember who I am, who my wife is, or what she had for breakfast that morning, but she takes care of her dog as if it was her child. During meal times, all she talks about with her friends is her dog, telling them how much she loves him (over and over, to the point that others probably wish she would stop!). Bear has changed her life, and both the dog's life and this lady's life are truly enriched for the pairing.

55 Gallons of Love

After college I decided to get a 55 gallon fish tank. I couldn't really tell you why I took on this project (tactic #24!), but I did. It took me several months of saving up, getting the parts, and figuring everything out, but the day I poured the fishies in was a pretty special day.

What I didn't realize at the time is how much I would enjoy watching my tank. Seeing the fish interact and go about their relatively meaningless lives was surprisingly relaxing. I later learned that while all pets are good for reducing stress, owning a fishtank in particular can actually lower your blood pressure.

Owning and operating the tank was time consuming and difficult at first, but sitting back and watching the tank was worth it. Putting a blue crayfish in the tank made the tank even more fun to watch. He would try to catch fish and fail, try to escape, and constantly move all of the tank's decorations around for no reason other than to mess things up.

I loved watching the tank and miss having one currently. I had to get rid of it for our move, but I do hope to start another one someday. My wife has been trying to convince me that we should get a dog so this chapter might be used against me in the near future!

How Pet Ownership Reduces Stress

Owning a pet is great for a good number of reasons, but one of the most beneficial is that it reduces our stress levels.

- Pets like dogs offer unconditional love to their owners. No matter how hard your day was, you are guaranteed that your dog will be happy to see you. Dogs don't judge you and always have your back!

- While we all need human connection from time to time, our relationships with our pets is not emotionally complicated. We can be ourselves around them no matter what!

- Pets give you a reason to keep on going even at your hardest times. No matter how hard your day was, you have to come home and take care of them.

- Having a solid routine keeps stress levels down by giving you a purpose day to day. You need to walk the dog in the morning, change the water in the fishtank, or give your cat some playtime. It gives you something to hold onto and something to look forward to each and every day.

- This doesn't really work for fish or porcupine owners (sorry!), but the physical contact of petting an animal can reduce blood pressure by lowering your heart rate. The act of petting the animal provides the opportunity for physical touch, which most of us need.

Practical Pet Ownership Tips

Here are several important tips on pet ownership and where to start if you want to get a pet!

1. Recognize that getting a pet is a huge commitment. Even my fish tank was a major commitment in that I had to constantly change the water and monitor everything. The level of commitment only increases if you decide to get a bigger animal like a dog or a cat.

2. Find someone you know that has an animal and ask them what it's like to own that animal. That will give you the best impression of what it's going to be like, and what to expect.

3. Figure out what type of pet you want. As I said above, you can even start with a plant if you really want to! Just be sure to spend a lot of time thinking and never buy a pet on impulse. That would be just plain stupid. If you change your mind, it isn't fair to you or the animal.

4. Research how to take care of the animal and purchase all the necessary gear. If you have a friend that has the type of animal you want, they will become your go-to person for advice.

5. Make sure you aren't allergic to the pet you want! I have bad allergies and will never be able to own a cat for this reason.

6. Be consistent and take care of the animal to the best of your ability. You'll find that your love for your pet will grow, and in time it will become part of your family.

Having a pet is an excellent way to give a home to an animal and to provide you with something that gives you a purpose beyond yourself. As with anything, there will be tough days (dog poop in the living room, anyone?), but in the end, getting a pet will enrich your life and provide you with a friendly and honorable companion.

Tactic #28: Get Rid of a Bad Habit!

This tactic is not for the faint of heart. It requires some serious motivation and willpower. However, accomplishing your weight loss goal will become much easier if you're able to get rid of a bad habit. The heavy burden of a bad habit will fall off of your shoulders, your stress levels will decline, and you'll feel light again.

Bad habits are part of the core reason why a lot of people struggle to lose weight, in that there are obstacles that are created by these bad habits. Stress levels rise as bad habits increase and flood our lives. The more obstacles we have, the more difficult and time consuming it is to see change occur.

Many of us have habits we're either too addicted, too lazy, too stubborn, or maybe even too scared to change. I challenge you take a good hard look at your life. Come up with a few reasons why your bad habits exist and why you struggle to defeat them. You need to be honest with yourself before change can occur.

Just a Few Bad Habits

None of the habits listed here are going to be earth shattering. Many of us deal with these bad habits daily, but don't worry, there is always hope! Here are several bad habits that you might be dealing with:

- Always reaching for dessert after every meal.
- Skipping breakfast.
- Eating right before bed.
- Forgetting to drink water throughout the day.
- Eating because you're upset.
- Staying up late to watch Netflix and thus not getting enough sleep.
- Watching too much TV, negatively affecting the brain.

- Buying junk food at the grocery store.

- Getting in debt.

- Eating fast food.

There are many bad habits out there, and your own may not have appeared on this list. However keep reading, as my own story and the practical tips I will share will give you hope that any bad habit can be overcome!

My Love of Soda

If you remember earlier in the book, I talked about how much I used to love soda. Growing up, I drank soda or juice more often than water. My bad habit was formed early on.

This continued into college, where having a can of Mountain Dew at least once a day was my norm. I loved drinking soda, and I would prefer a can for lunch, supper, and a snack if I could convince myself that I deserved it.

It was clear that this habit was unhealthy, but the fact that I needed to get rid of it never took a firm grasp in my mind. It took many years for me to overcome my love of soda and be rid of it forever. I did reduce my intake dramatically when I started my weight loss journey, but I still had it on the weekends and every once in awhile during the week. I still lost weight. Drinking soda wasn't the end of the world. But part of me knew that I should be doing more, and that I WAS capable of doing more.

I'm proud to say that as of August 12th, 2015 I have been soda free; I have not had ANY since then. It was a choice I made after leaving a leadership summit. The summit was a 2 day event that left me with a renewed sense of determination. The event focuses on preparing individuals for leadership, but also seeks to change leaders in their own lives.

Craig Groeschel, senior pastor at Life Church, was one of the speakers at the event. His message was excellent, and the overall point was that we are capable of more than we realize. I left feeling like I needed to step up my game and enrich my life in some way. It was obvious to me that drinking soda was just an unnecessary and unhealthy bad habit, so I decided to nix it.

It was a difficult decision, and yet it wasn't. If you truly believe in yourself and take a stand, you can do anything you put your mind to. We're capable of so much more than we know, and our potential is beyond what we could even imagine.

What do you love that you could get rid of?

What habit do you have that just isn't good for you?

Overcome Bad Habits to Reach Freedom

There are varying levels of difficulty with breaking habits. As I stated earlier, smoking is a particularly nasty habit because of its addictive nature, making it difficult to quit by willpower alone. Still, I'm convinced that any bad habit can be put to rest if you have the grit and determination to see it through.

Here are some practical ways to eliminate a bad habit from your life:

1. The first step in eliminating a bad habit is to pick one. Have a lot of bad habits? Focus on one at a time and change slowly. Prioritize which ones affect you the most negatively, and destroy those habits first.

2. Tell a loved one (or the world!) that you're attempting to break your habit. Don't be afraid to share, as many others probably have a similar bad habit, and their own journeys may be bolstered by your resolve. You'll be empowered knowing that you've made a public commitment to breaking the habit.

3. Take it one day at a time. Whatever the habit is, make changes daily to reach your goal. Have a smaller amount of soda, eat half a donut, or remember to drink water in the morning.

4. Replace your bad habit with another activity. Avoid boredom at all costs!

5. Figure out when you're most likely to lose motivation. Do whatever you can to avoid making a bad choice in a vulnerable moment.

6. One of the most important steps to remember is that you're only human. You might have times that your willpower collapses and you give in. Don't beat yourself up; just pick yourself up and go at it with a renewed sense of determination.

7. Never give up! At all costs figure out a way to break your bad habit!

Tactic #29: Drink Tea

According to archeological evidence, tea drinking has been around for quite some time. It most likely originated in China and spread from there, eventually becoming popular in countries like Great Britain where tea time was a common occurrence. Nowadays you can find tea in any grocery store in many flavors and varieties.

Tea reduces stress, is full of antioxidants, and it can help prevent many different diseases. Tea drinking is the superhero secret sauce when it comes to being crazy healthy. Say goodbye to energy drinks or espresso shot power ups. Drink tea instead to fuel your engines and wave goodbye to health issues.

For the most benefit from tea stick to the four main types that derive from the camellia sinensis plant. Herbal teas have their benefits, but for the most part it is better to stick to these types:

- Green Tea

- Black Tea

- White Tea

- Oolong Tea

In this chapter I will discuss Green and black teas as these are the most common varieties; white and oolong teas account for less than 1% of all tea production and sales in the world.

Green Tea

Green tea is one of the most commonly known kind of teas. If asked if green tea was good for them, most people would probably say "yeah of course!" But the reality is that only 50% of Americans are drinking tea every day (according to Calorie Lab), and only a small portion of those tea drinkers are drinking green tea.

Where to find it: You can get green tea in stores via tea bags or bottle. Be careful buying a jug of green tea though, as some brands may have added sugar to it. As I talked about with tactic #10 (reducing added sugars) there is no reason to get a good thing going if it means adding sugar to your diet.

A major health benefit: Green tea is an amazing stress reducer due to its high level of antioxidants. In addition, another active component in green tea called epigallocatechin gallate aids in reducing physical and mental fatigue.

Black Tea

Black tea is more oxidized than the other teas listed here and has a strong, unique flavor. It's the most common tea in the world, for about 90% of the global tea trade.

Where to find it: Black tea is commonly found in iced teas or tea bags. It has many different varieties and flavors. The most common varieties are Lipton, Earl Gray, and English Breakfast tea. As with green tea, watch out for too much added sugar!

A major health benefit: Studies have proven that black tea can help your teeth by limiting plaque build up and controlling bacteria in the mouth.

How Green Tea Helped Me to Reduce Stress at Work

When work gets really busy and you're responsible for a lot of things, stress ensues. It's the natural way of things. We know we need to reduce stress in order to avoid health problems. Yet eliminating what causes our stress is often impossible. Sure, I could have quit my job, but how many jobs these days don't create extra stress? Let me know if you find a good one for me!

I was becoming so stressed during the day I could feel my stomach tightening. I called it a "stress pit." I was in the midst of eating healthier and exercising regularly, but no matter what I did, work was always there to make my gut feel terrible.

I wasn't sure what the next step was, so I did some research. I came upon green tea and boy am I glad I did! I drank it hot by microwaving water in a mug and then steeping a teabag in it. I started drinking at least two cups of green tea every afternoon and my symptoms improved greatly. I felt an immediate difference in my stomach. I made sure to drink as much green tea as possible during meetings, while on the phone, and doing reports. Drinking green tea made a huge difference and greatly reduced the stress pit in my stomach.

To this day I still drink green tea often, as I find that it improves my mood and keeps stress at bay. Tea drinking is an easy and practical step towards improving how you feel from day to day.

Easy Ways to Drink More Tea

1. Drinking more tea is not complicated at all. Follow these tips to get more tea into your diet:

2. Replace soda or juice with hot tea. Tea has a great flavor and is a better choice hands down than the sugary alternatives.

3. Hungry at night? Have a cup of decaf tea to avoid eating too much too late.

4. Mix tea into a smoothie instead of plain water. This way you can get the benefits of tea without having to taste it.

5. Try different varieties and flavors of green and black tea in order to keep things interesting.

6. Remember that everything in moderation applies to tea as well. Going from 0 cups per day to 15 could really mess with your system.

Tactic #30: Listen to Music

Unless you live out in the woods with no electricity, you're pretty much guaranteed to listen to some sort of music each and every day. Whether you're a jazz fan or prefer rock and roll, there is a music genre out there for you.

Many people go to music for stress reduction when they don't even realize it. Others listen solely during a workout to distract their minds from the grueling task at hand. Some people listen in their cars and rock out during their cruise down the highway. It doesn't matter where you listen; the important thing is to keep listening!

The next time you reach for a bottle of beer to relax a bit after a hard day's work, why not try sitting down, putting your feet up, and listening to some calming music instead? You might find that your mind is more at ease and the music reduces your stress much better than alcohol.

My Favorite Music

My favorite band is Owl City. The lead singer, Adam Young, sings to electronic background music. His music sends a calm over my mind, and it causes me to feel grounded.

I don't branch out all that much with music. I enjoy listening to Owl City songs over and over again. That's just my preference, and I really don't think there is any right or wrong way to go about it. If heavy metal resonates with you, then by all means go ahead and listen to them. But if heavy metal causes you stress, as it certainly would do to me and other people, don't listen to it.

I listen to music while writing, while I'm at the gym, and while driving. I don't listen as much as other people might, but I can certainly attest to the fact that listening to music reduces my stress levels. Listening to a worship song, or listening to the rhythmic tunes of Owl City certainly does my mind good!

How Music Reduces Stress

In one study music was shown to reduce anxiety symptoms in patients before and after surgery. Due to listening to music patients required less pain medication post surgery. These findings are huge when considering how we can reduce stress, because music is basically free to listen to.

Another study was done to measure the effects of music on several women who were given stress tests. The women who listened to relaxing music during the stressful situations displayed a lower stress response to the external stimuli. The study was inconclusive, but it did demonstrate that listening to music has an effect on the brain.

Certain types of music are also extremely helpful for meditation, which is excellent news if you're trying tactic #26 (meditation). Music eases your mind and prevents your thoughts from wandering this way and that. It's especially helpful to pair worship music with prayer as the music keeps your mind focused on what is most important.

I can't say exactly what music is capable of in your life, because we're all very different and have very different tastes! The best judge is you and how you feel. It's up to you to find the music that works for you.

Practical and Fun Ways To Fill Your Life With Music

Here are some tips to enjoying music more often! You might already do a lot of these already, but there is no reason to not add a little bit more music to your life!

1. One great tip from healthguide.org is to wake up in the morning to the music of your choice. It's a good way to slowly ease into your day. You can hear one of your favorite songs instead of an annoying news report or the BLAP BLAP BLAP of an alarm clock!

2. Playing or singing along with music is a great way to challenge your-self as well as have fun. I used to play the trumpet in high school, and I truly believe that doing so was one of the main reasons I did well in school. My band teacher always said that being in band made

us better students. Reading and playing music trains your mind to fire certain brain synapses.

3. Listen to music while walking, running, or even lifting. It will pump you up and get you ready to knock out a solid workout.

4. Listen to music when you're in the car. Music can soothe the symptoms of road rage that appear in even the nicest people.

Like to cook? Put on some music while you mix up those ingredients. This way, you can dance and burn some extra calories before you eat the delicious food you're making.

Section 5

TACTICS FOR PRACTICAL APPLICATION

Conference calls at work can be the worst. Listening to your boss criticize you and all of your fellow co-workers never feels good. In fact, it can feel downright miserable. All you hear is, "We need to get better at A!" and "Make sure that you remember to do B!" And "Blah, blah, blah." You leave the meeting thinking:

1. "I learned nothing from that."

2. "That was a waste of time."

3. "What was it even about?"

I hear you saying, "Why would you bring this up? I was almost stress free after the last section!"

Throughout this book I have given you several weight loss tactics, each with their own tips to apply the tactics in a practical way. While each tactic on its own will definitely improve your life, you'll need an extra push to reach your goals and make lifelong changes.

There needs to be a boss that not only tells you what to do but *how* to do it. She needs to be able to tell you that you need to get from point A to B by doing this, this, and then that. It doesn't do any good if she screams at you to "Sell more paper!" if you don't have any idea how to actually sell paper.

Practical application is where the rubber meets the road. It's where you say "Okay self, let's get going." It's where you put all of your hard-won knowledge into action.

Knowing about weight loss doesn't do you any good if you don't know how to put it into action. In this section I'll discuss four tactics for making your dream a reality. These tactics will push your journey to a new level.

These final four tactics encompass goal setting, taking steps to reach those goals, keeping track of your progress, and keeping yourself accountable by getting an accountability partner.

Mastering these tactics will help you to realize true success in the form of life change that sticks. No longer will you lose hope in a diet, or succumb to the pull of a bad habit, because you've armed yourself to fight back.

With these handy application tactics, you'll be able to have the body you've always wanted, and the positive habits you'll form will change your life for years to come.

"My philosophy of life is that if we make up our mind what we are going to make of our lives, then work hard toward that goal, we never lose — somehow we always win out." ~ Ronald Reagan

---

Tactic #31: Set a Crazy and Insane Weight Loss Goal

Reaching your desired weight is not an easy process, nor does it happen overnight. However, you can more easily overcome the day-to-day drag by setting a major goal for yourself. This crazy goal has to be very specific. It needs to have:

1. A specific starting point

2. A desired end point

3. When you'll reach your goal

For example, your fitness/weight loss goal could be any of the following:

- I'm going to go from 220 pounds to 175 pounds by 6/16/16.

- I will go from running 5 miles a week to 25 miles a week by 6/16/16.

- I will go from a BMI of 30 to 20 by 6/16/16.

Any of these goals will work because they are for a specific time frame, and they are measurable. When 6/16/16 comes around you'll know for 100% certain whether or not you achieved your goal. There will be no wiggle room and no ambiguity. It forces you to work towards your goal and it gives you a burning passion to do so.

The goal needs to be achievable and realistic, but it also needs to be EPIC. When you reach your goal you'll want to shout your success from the rooftops (or post about it on Facebook!).

Where do you want to see yourself in 6 months?

How would it feel if you had done something difficult and amazing and you'd totally changed your life?

What would it be like to have lost the weight and achieved victory?

How much better off do you think you could be if you buckled down and really fought hard to reach your goal?

When I was first losing weight I didn't set a specific goal. My road would have been so much easier had I set a crazy goal for myself right from the start. I would have seen that in no time at all I could achieve what I thought was a ridiculous goal, and that I could soar much higher than I knew.

I didn't lose the weight quickly. It took months before I started to see any change. Had I been tracking and working towards a weight goal, I would have been able to reach my ideal weight much faster. I would have been able to see where I was going, what I had to do, and how much time I had to get there.

I recently set a goal for completing this book. I would have it completely written by the end of February of 2016. I would go from 10 chapters to 35 by 2/29/16. I would have the first draft finished and ready to be edited. I made this goal in January and I figured I would have plenty of time to reach it.

Naturally, February rolled around and I wasn't even close to being on target for a February completion date. Yikes! I would have to buckle down; failure was not an option. I put my rear in gear, scheduled out how many chapters I would have to do every night, and I was able to reach my goal with a few days to spare!

The power of setting goals is incredible. Setting a weight loss goal is important for self-motivation. Decide you're going to do something and do not let yourself down. If you want to be more active, more fit, and happier with your body, then you need to set a goal to make it happen. Just one day at the gym or one day of eating healthy will NOT cut it.

The hard truth is that change only happens when you're committed to making small changes each and every day to better yourself for the long term. Each day you need to reach for your goal. You have the power within yourself to rise up and smash your goal into little tiny pieces. You can and will reach your goal by a certain time frame.

Follow these steps to picking a goal:

1. Make sure the goal is specific in the final results. This is so important because the goal needs to be trackable and you need to know how you're doing at any given point. If you're one month in, haven't lost any weight, and it doesn't look like you'll reach your goal, you can change course and quickly figure out what you're doing wrong. You also need to know WHEN you finally reach it so you can celebrate!

2. Make the goal EPIC as well as possible. You can't have six pack abs in two weeks, but you can do much more than lose 10 pounds in a year.

3. Research your ideal weight and decide how long it will take you to get there.

4. You can be as creative as you want with this goal. Choosing to lift a certain amount or run a certain distance are great goals, because more than likely everything else will follow suit. If you work hard to achieve the goal of running a half marathon, then there is a good chance you'll purposely eat better too in order to reach that goal, which will help to lose weight.

5. Don't get completely stuck on what the scale says. Some of us are bigger boned that other people, OR we like to weight lift and thus have more muscle. The real goal should be to eat healthier and be able to live a life free of the many ailments that overweight people face.

Pick a goal that is just right for you, and follow it up with the next tactic to crush that goal into oblivion.

The Fiber Guardian muttered quietly to himself "I will destroy Lacka-daisical and master all 35 tactics by the end of this year." A goal had been placed, the flag planted, and the course set. He was so close he could taste sweet victory like the honey from a fresh beehive. Only laziness and fear of failure could stop him now!

Tactic #32: Take Action and Choose your Tactics!

Bradley Whitford (an actor most recently seen in Brooklyn 99 as Jake Peralta's father) sums up action-taking perfectly:

"Infuse your life with action. Don't wait for it to happen. Make it happen. Make your own future. Make your own hope. Make your own love. And whatever your beliefs, honor your creator, not by passively waiting for grace to come down from upon high, but by doing what you can to make grace happen… yourself, right now, right down here on Earth."

This is what *The Action Diet* is all about! Conquering goals with determined and focused action. This action must be accomplished daily and without pause in a consistent fashion. You can wait for things to happen to you, or you can take action today and make things happen.

The old maxim of "good things come to those who wait" might be good for those who need to learn patience, but it's a phrase that too many have taken literally. One day I will meet my spouse, one day I will write a book, one day I will lose weight, one day… but "one day" might never come. Change will not happen until you make changes in your life. You have to make the choice for yourself to make changes.

I recognize that for many of you the journey seems daunting and even starting feels overwhelming. Please don't mistake my honesty here for an attempt to put you down. I know how hard it can be; but I also know that there's only one person that can make a change in your life, and that someone is YOU.

Choosing the right tactics

I recognize that incorporating all of the tactics in this book isn't easy. It's not probable to take every single tactic and work it into your life in weeks. It took me years to master all of these tactics and to incorporate them into my own life.

It's imperative that you choose the right tactics that are going to work for you. Pick the tactics that you think are fun. If you HATE walking, then tactic #17 is not going to work for you.

I suggest picking a tactic from each major group (food related, exercise, and stress reduction tactics), along with the first two tactics, and start there. it's best to keep things simple, especially when you're just starting out.

Here are three sample tactic groups that you can begin to use right away to start to see results and to make a positive change in your life.

Starting out sample A:

- Focus (tactic #1)
- Water consumption (tactic #2)
- Focus on fiber (tactic #4)
- Walk everywhere (tactic #16)
- Find a Project (tactic #24)

Starting out sample B:

- Focus (tactic #1)
- Water consumption (tactic #2)
- Increase protein intake (tactic #10)
- Lift (tactic #18)
- Drink Tea (tactic #29)

Starting out sample C:

- Focus (tactic #1)
- Water consumption (tactic #2)
- Drink Coffee (tactic #14)
- Interval training (tactic #19)
- Get rid of a bad habit (tactic #28)

If you're not sure where to begin, start out with one of these groups as your main set of tactics. Use these tactics every day and see how you do with them. As you master the groups of tactics you can add others into your arsenal.

The armory was unlocked and the Fiber Guardian walked in. Along the wall he saw tactics of all different forms and sizes. Now fully understanding, he reached out and grasped what appeared to a water goblet and a medallion that resembled a brain. He was immediately infused with radiant power and lightning sparked around him. Striding further into the compound he found a pair of walking shoes with his "FG" symbol imbued upon them, as well a coffee mug that was similarly inscribed. With one final glance at all of his other choices of weaponry, he snagged a pair of green headphones. He then confidently began walking to meet his arch nemesis and defeat him once and for all.

Tactic #33: Create a Scoreboard to Track your Progress

What would the NFL be like if we didn't have a way to keep track of the score of the game? What if no one kept score and the teams just played for the love of the game? What if the team members all sat around a fire afterward singing Kumbaya without a care for who won or lost?

To most people, this suggestion feels like a nail scraping across a chalkboard. The idea of a scoreless game is ridiculous. What would be the point of playing? Why would anyone bother watching?

Football would not be what it is today if there wasn't a clear winner and loser. We're able to tell which team is winning or losing just by glancing at a scoreboard. The NFL scoreboard shows you which quarter you're in, how much time is left, the down, how many yards to go, and the overall score. All of this information makes it easy to keep track of the game by showing the players where they are going.

For our own practical use, a scoreboard is a great way to keep track of our goals and quickly see whether we are winning or losing. It keeps us accountable and keeps us heading in the right direction—if the scoreboard has the right components.

The Components of a Great Scoreboard

A scoreboard needs the right components to be an asset to your weight loss journey. Here are the most important factors to remember:

1. Score with your personality in mind: The scoreboard can be on the medium of your choice, whether digital or paper. If you like a good smartphone app, then go for it. If you want to make the scoreboard a huge poster and plaster it up on the wall, that's great too. You can make a spreadsheet, use sticky notes, or keep score on your bath-

room mirror with a glass marker. As long as the scoreboard is visual and will keep you coming back to update it, it works.

2. Keep it visible: It needs to be visible to you. This means that if it's on your phone, you need to be driven to look at it once in awhile (through reminders or placing it on the home screen). If it's an actual physical scoreboard it needs to be somewhere you'll see it every day.

3. Keep it simple: Anyone looking at the scoreboard has to quickly see if you're winning or losing. Too much data will make this difficult.

4. Include the goal and the tactics you have chosen. These need to be present on the scoreboard because you'll be updating it constantly in order to effectively track your progress.

A Sample Scoreboard

A good scoreboard for weight loss will display the goal as the biggest, most visible part of the scoreboard. It will have the tactics within easy view. You will be forced to look at it at least daily, but you'll enjoy looking at. You'll be able to tell exactly where you are in your goal progress at a glance.

See the picture below for a sample weight loss scoreboard. It includes 5 tactics from this book and has all of the components of a successful scoreboard.

As you can see in this scoreboard the goal weight and the starting weight are clearly present. It is simple and you can easily track your progress as you go along. Also listed are the tactics that are going to move you along with your goal.

SCOREBOARD

MARCH 2015 → AUGUST 2015

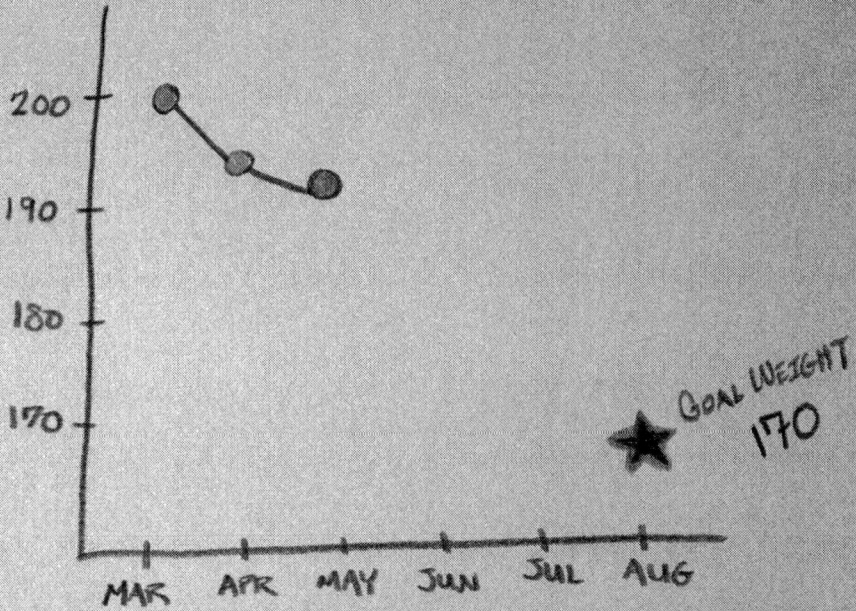

200
190
180
170

GOAL WEIGHT
170

MAR   APR   MAY   JUN   JUL   AUG

Focus

★ DRINK MORE WATER
★ WALK EVERYWHERE
★ FIND A PROJECT
★ EAT MORE FIBER

Why Having a Scoreboard is Important

At the end of the day, tracking your progress toward a goal is monumental in the successful completion of that goal. I tracked every chapter I wrote in this book, and it would have taken me much longer to complete it if I hadn't been tracking my progress on a scoreboard that I placed on the wall. It looked like a simple checklist, but it kept me accountable and helped me to finish on time.

A scoreboard keeps your goal a reality from day to day. It keeps your goal at the forefront of your mind and keeps you accountable to your success. Updating it daily or weekly keeps the attention on the goal and allows you to make adjustments if needed. It shows you what's working and what's not. If you find that a particular tactic isn't working for you, you can update the scoreboard to reflect that change.

A scoreboard is a means of staying consistent and accountable. But accountability is easier when you have someone else to help you out.

Tactic #34 Find an Accountability Partner

If you hang out with chickens, you're going to cluck and if you hang out with eagles, you're going to fly. — Steve Maraboli

D o you want to just cluck around or do you want to soar?

Finding an accountability partner will lead you to success. This person will keep you up when you're down, and will push you to that next level when you need it. With the perfect partner judgment never plays a role; as your partner will never put you down, nor will they be jealous of your accomplishments.

My Accountability Partner

In my own life, my wife is my accountability partner. She pushes me to reach my goals, updates my scoreboard if I forget, and will change my goal if she doesn't think it's "crazy" enough. She is my rock and she is the reason I have come as far as I have.

I firmly believe that we weren't meant to go through life alone. We weren't meant to struggle alone, nor were we meant to celebrate on our own. I have experienced these truths first hand because I have celebrated success with my wife, but we have also struggled through failure.

Together we have enjoyed the good moments and the bad, and I know that I couldn't do it without her. I could not have lost the weight after college. I could not have quit my job and moved hundreds of miles away without her, and I would not have ever been able to finish this book without her.

Finding someone that supports you unconditionally may not be easy, but there are ways to find yourself a good partner.

How to Find an Accountability Partner

A good accountability partner won't drop from the sky and be ready for action. However, recognize that just about everyone has a goal they would like to reach and you can offer to be their accountability partner in exchange for their help.

Here are a few practical steps to finding an accountability partner:

1. Make a list of possible people you can ask to be your partner. Any of the following might be good options, but only you can decide who the best person is:

   • Your spouse

   • A sibling

   • A parent

   • A gym trainer

   • A good friend

   • A co-worker

2. Choose a person that will be tough on you when you need it most, but also someone that will pick you up when you're feeling down.

3. Pick someone that is close enough to you to know what you need to hear when you need to hear it.

4. Pick someone who can check in with you at least once a week to see how you're doing with your goals.

No accountability partner will be perfect. They won't always say the perfect thing, but the point is that they're on your side. At the end of the day they're on your team and will see that you reach your goals, one way or another.

Qualities of the Perfect Accountability Arrangement

The following are a few qualities of a good accountability partnership:

• Competition – In the words of the great professor Keating from the movie Dead Poet's Society-"Sports are a chance for other human beings to push us to excel." Other people have the capacity to push us to excel, especially when we're competitive! If you're in competition with your partner, things can progress quickly, as you're both trying to outdo one another!

- Honesty and Trust – The moment "one bite of blueberry pie" actually means that you downed the entire pie can spell disaster for your accountability partnership. Trusting your partner is hugely important. It will make it much more difficult to be honest with your person if they make fun of you or bad mouth you to others.

- Belief in your success – Your partner must believe that you can succeed, and you must also believe in their success. Any doubts that you have about each other will seep in like a poison. This poison will ultimately destroy the partnership and neither of you will find success.

In the end, having an accountability partner will keep you focused on the tactics and it will move you in the right direction towards your goals. With the right amount of determination you'll both find success in whatever goals you have!

The Protein Kapow and The Fiber Guardian called Lackadaisical out from behind his lazy boy. The arena was set and the battle began, there is no room for monologues in this story! As the Fiber Guardian walked toward Lackadaisical he heard The Protein Kapow cheering him on, telling him that he could indeed win the war!

The Fiber Guardian struck first, spraying water all over Lackadaisical creating a loud hissing sound as Lackadaisical was burned by the touch of water. The enemy shook off the hit and calmly lowered his left hand palm facing up. With the other hand he conjured a succulent Krispy Kreme donut and placed it on his open palm.

The Fiber Guardian stopped in his tracks. This was it… This was the ultimate choice. He hesitated for only a second and then took a bite of his own apple instead. Lackadaisical roared in horror at this unexpected turn of events and he ran off into the night, with FG hot on his heels to finish the war once and for all.

Tactic #35: Constantly Evaluate Your Status

One of the most important tactics that I used during my weight loss journey was to constantly reevaluate my status and to make changes where appropriate. This tactic encourages you to stop, think, and adjust your lifestyle as needed in order to continue making progress.

Too often we find ourselves in a rut and don't take steps to get out of the rut. There was one time in particular that I had started to creep back up in my weight. I was flabbergasted as to what the cause could be. I thought I was doing everything right. (I was only really doing "okay")

I felt like I was moving in the right direction, but my choices of food were growing stale, and I was becoming bored with my new diet. I ate donuts more often, binged on candy, and ate dessert almost every day. I was bored and needed to take a step back. I needed to take action and make yet another series of changes.

At the time I didn't think, "Wow, I really need to use tactic #35 and reevaluate my current status!" But I did see that I was losing every step I'd gained.

Failure is not an option in my book. I wasn't going to lose sight of the end goal. I wasn't going to give up. I was finally on my way to getting in shape and I wouldn't be stopped, damnit!

It was the first time that I fully reevaluated, and it wouldn't be the last.

This re-eval started with a trip to the grocery store, where I decided that fruit smoothies would be the way to go. These smoothies did more than just cause me to begin losing weight again.

Steps to Reevaluate

The following are the steps that I took to refocus and obtain new direction and passion for losing weight.

1. Find something new: Research new foods to try and plan new meals. Find a new sport or physical activity that you like to do. Doing something new is a great way to start fresh and get excited about weight loss.

2. Try it: Go to the grocery store and buy the new foods and meal ingredients. Toss the frisbee around with a friend or join their league. Even if you think you might not fall in love with it you should give it a try.

3. Set a trial period: Make the current week a trial week and try several new foods and activities during this time. This will give you renewed hope that you're heading in the right direction.

4. Be honest with yourself. You know how you have been doing better than anyone. If you ate horribly and sat around and watched TV all day admit your folly and move on. You have the ability to recognize what you need to change in order to see progress.

5. Do NOT beat yourself up over past mistakes. Don't think that because you failed in the past that means you will fail again. It only works that way if you believe that it will so believe in yourself! Believe that you will make better decisions from here on out and forget what came before.

6. Have fun with it! Try new foods or activities that you think you might enjoy. It's not about choking down kale salads and beet pudding or going on long runs if that isn't your thing. It's about making foods that you find that are simultaneously delicious and nutritious, and about finding something active that you love to do.

7. Take action. It is not enough to read about it and not take a step forward. Stop telling yourself that it is too hard or too painful. Tell yourself that you can do it and that you will do it. Take that step forward in order to come out on top.

Following these steps takes determination and a will to defeat any boredom that is growing from your choices. However, it's a tactic that reinvigorates you to be able to complete your goal.

Take that step back, ponder. reevaluate, and ultimately you'll conquer and crush your goals into oblivion! You will find that doing so is one of the best decisions you'll ever make.

As he runs away Lackadaisical knows that he has one one final miniscule ray of hope that he can find victory… He will hide away and wait for FG to lose motivation! Certainly that will work! But then… NO it cannot be, the Fiber Guardian steps around the corner holding the mirror of truth. FG knows the secret now. As long as he continually looks upon himself in honesty he will never again face defeat.

Lackadaisical feels himself drifting away. He has no place in this world anymore. He has been defeated and is banished forever. The Fiber Guardian has won the war and has leveled up to superhero status once and for all!

Closing Thoughts

Reaching your desired weight will not happen overnight. It takes a good while before you begin to see change. It does not happen quickly enough for most people to be happy with the results. That's why most diets fail; people do not stick with them long enough, or were given false promises as to how quickly they would lose the weight ("Lose 10 pounds in 10 days! Blast fat in a matter of minutes!").

I hope you've found that *The Action Diet* made no false promises or suggested that weight loss would be easy. The tactics themselves are easy enough, but seeing results takes hard work, motivation, and a new level of determination. It requires taking action!

Trust me on this next point though: once you start to get into your new routine, focusing on tactical groups, the weight will start to fall off. When I started my journey it was rough at first, with plenty of downs mixed in with the ups. But eventually I started to lose weight continuously, and the compliments flooded my way from family members, friends, and co-workers.

It took a doctor telling me that I needed to lose weight for me to take action. The doctor's words could have been much worse than just a friendly suggestion. Had I continued on the path I was on, my path back to health would have been that much more difficult. I wrote this book and shared these tactics so you that you can avoid the mistakes I made, and have more success, more quickly than I did.

Remember the practical steps to find success and apply these to your own journey:

1. Make a crazy big goal

2. Choose your tactics

3. Keep track of your progress

4. Stay on the right path by getting an accountability partner

5. Continue to make changes and evaluate your current situation

I'm certain you can find success as I did if you incorporate these tactics into your daily life. I'm confident that you can do it, no matter your age or your abilities. Anyone can make a life-changing decision if they have the hustle and the grit required to do so.

Are you ready to get gritty?

Are you ready to apply what you've learned?

Are you ready to see change within your own life?

I think you're ready, and I know that you can do it. Now get going.

If you've found this book helpful and my insights pleasureable, I suggest that you sign up for my mailing list by going here (http://bit.ly/1RrmguU).

I will send you frequent tips on weight loss and how to stay focused on your goals.

For even more immediate information, check out my website at www.Fiberguardian.com. I share all about the high fiber diet and how to best incorporate high fiber foods into your daily eating habits. I also respond to any questions from my fans. While I'm not a doctor or health professional by any means, I can surely help you get started by pointing you in the right direction.

Thank you so much for reading this book, and good luck with your own weight loss adventure!

-Jordan, Your Fiber Guardian

For further reading on losing weight, I suggest the following books:

1. *Level Up Your Life: How to Unlock Adventure and Happiness by Becoming the Hero of Your Own Story* By Steve Kamb

2. *It Starts With Food: Discover the Whole30 and Change Your Life in Unexpected Ways* By Dallas and Melissa Hartwig

3. *How to Eat, Move and Be Healthy!* By Paul Chek

4. *Exercise Every Day: 32 Tactics for Building the Exercise Habit (Even If You Hate Working Out)* By S. J. Scott

Before You Go...

If you enjoyed reading this book I would very much appreciate a positive review. Reviews will help my book climb the rankings and ultimately reach more people!

Thank you for supporting an indie author!

About the Author

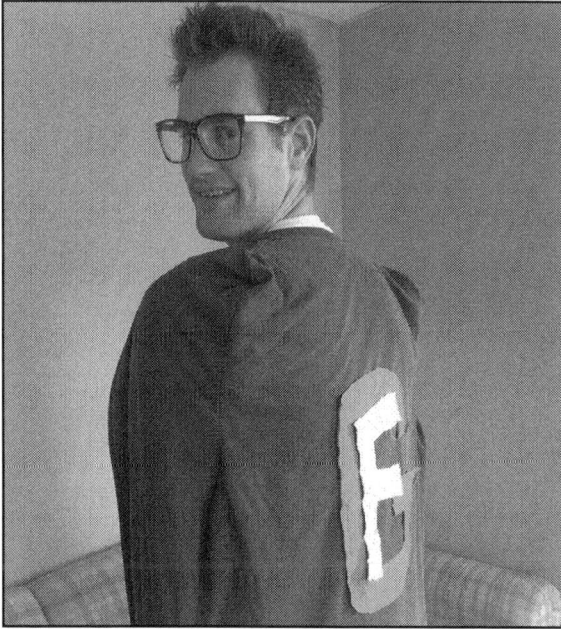

Jordan Ring is the owner and creator of <u>Fiberguardian.com</u>. He enjoys making weird faces, doing ridiculous Fiber Guardian videos, eating apples, and playing ultimate frisbee with his wife. He is obsessed with the high fiber diet and is currently in the best shape of his life and enjoying every minute of it. He believes in taking action and taking accountability for his own choices, and has made it a life goal to share his ideas with the world.

Manufactured by Amazon.ca
Bolton, ON